EXPERTS' PRAISE FOR DR. JOHN R. LEE'S BOOK AND THE RESULTS OF HIS NATURAL PROGESTERONE THERAPY!

"With a penetrating eye for truth and a courageous disregard for self-interest, John Lee makes clear sense out of the confusing area of women's hormone therapy. In the process he demonstrates the best remedy for our health care crisis: a physician whose first priority is the patient's welfare."

—*Philip Incao, M.D., family practice physician*

"Natural progesterone has been an important, exciting, and innovative addition to my wellness practice in women's health care. It is a strategic part of my treatment of PMS, menopause, osteoporosis, irregular menses, fibrocystic breasts, endometriosis, and more. I no longer have use for the unnatural Provera and other progestins that cause so many unnecessary side effects. Now that we have begun to realize the dangers of environmental chemicals that mimic estrogen, I am even more grateful to discover that natural progesterone helps to safely restore healthy hormone balance."

—*Jesse Hanley, M.D., director, Malibu Health and Rehabilitation*

"A must-read for every woman over forty who wants to avoid the dangers of synthetic hormone replacement therapy."

—*Dr. Earl Mindell, author of* **The Vitamin Bible**

more...

AND WOMEN AGREE!

"After ten years on Premarin and Provera, I took the initiative to discontinue all synthetic hormones and tried natural progesterone. My symptoms were less the first month, even less the second month, and the third month was a breeze! No symptoms at all. I didn't retain water, craving for sweets was not noticeable, breast problems were gone, and best of all, no sinus headache."

—H.A., *Norcross, GA*

"Thank you for your work: for being concerned about women's bones, for not believing that osteoporosis is irreversible....My bones are delighted, so is my hormone balance, and so is my husband!"

—S.S., *San Diego, CA*

"For years I searched for a doctor who believed there was a correlation between my headaches, allergies, etc., and my hormonal imbalance. I am very grateful for your book, your research, and your time."

—T.T., *Moraga, CA*

"I spent three years with migraine headaches, terrible aches in my pelvis, severe fatigue, severe memory loss and sometimes complete disorientation, terrific depression, and I had cold- and flu-like symptoms constantly. I tried everything. It wasn't until a friend of mine introduced me to natural progesterone that things changed. In one month every symptom went away. My life has changed in a big way. It's a godsend."

—V.S., *Novato, CA*

WHAT YOUR DOCTOR MAY *NOT* TELL YOU

ABOUT

MENOPAUSE

THE BREAKTHROUGH BOOK ON *NATURAL* PROGESTERONE

JOHN R. LEE, M.D.

WITH VIRGINIA HOPKINS

WARNER BOOKS

A Time Warner Company

Grateful acknowledgment is given for permission to quote from the following: Copyright *Physicians' Desk Reference,* 1994, 48th edition, published by Medical Economics Company, Montvale, New Jersey 07645. Reprinted by permission. All rights reserved.

Publisher's Note:

The information in this book can be a valuable addition to your doctor's advice, but it is not intended to replace the services of trained health professionals. You are advised to consult with your health care professional with regard to matters relating to your health, and in particular regarding symptoms that may require diagnosis or immediate attention.

Warner Books, Inc., 1271 Avenue of the Americas, New York, NY 10020

 A Time Warner company

Printed in the United States of America
First Printing: May 1996
10 9 8 7 6 5 4 3 2

Library of Congress Cataloging-in-Publication Data
Lee, John R., M.D.
    What your doctor may not tell you about menopause : the breakthrough book on natural progesterone / John R. Lee with Virginia Hopkins.
        p. cm.
    Includes index.
    ISBN 0-446-67144-4
    1. Menopause—Hormone therapy. 2. Progesterone—Therapeutic use. 3. Menopause—Complications—Alternative treatment. I. Hopkins, Virginia. II. Title.
RG186.L44
618.1'75061—dc20   95-44748
                                                              CIP

Book design by Charles Sutherland
Cover design by Rachel McClain

CONTENTS

FOREWORD

I first heard of natural progesterone seventeen years ago. Twenty-three years out of medical school and in my twentieth year of family practice in Mill Valley, California, I had been invited to present a report on hypoglycemia to the Orthomolecular Medical Society in San Francisco. After giving my paper, I returned to the audience to listen to the next presentation, a talk by Ray Peat, Ph.D., of Oregon. His subject was natural progesterone, its many roles in human health, and a criticism of the medical profession for having ignored this important hormone in the care of women's health. As I recall, Dr. Peat argued that giving unopposed estrogen (estrogen replacement without progesterone) to women after menopause was, in short, the wrong thing to be doing. The force of his argument, the scientific knowledge he laid out, and the references he provided were a clear challenge to the prevailing practice of most of us in the room. We had all been taught that menopause (when the ovaries stopped making their hormones) led to a variety of female complaints that represented estrogen deficiency. We had believed it obvious to treat such patients with estrogen. Yet here was a Ph.D. in biochemistry telling us we were wrong.

Taking the opportunity to snare Dr. Peat immediately after his talk, I spent the next hour or so with him exploring the subject further and getting his list of references. In the months that followed,

I read as many of the papers he had listed as I could find. The evidence was strong that Dr. Peat was right: Giving estrogen alone just did not make good sense. In the process of this research, I came upon more and more evidence that not only was progesterone an important hormone at all adult ages for both men and women but also that unopposed estrogen put women at risk of undesirable, potentially lethal side effects.

Just a year or so before, it had become evident that women using estrogen were at five to six times greater risk of endometrial cancer (cancer of the uterus) than women not using estrogen. In effect, women and their doctors had to make a cruel choice between using estrogen to prevent osteoporosis and increase their risk of uterine cancer or not using it and risk an earlier hip fracture. Further, many of my women patients on estrogen had experienced water retention, headaches, and tender, swollen breasts, in addition to becoming fatter no matter how they dieted.

The turning point came for me when I was confronted with patients I had known for years who now had progressive osteoporosis and could not take estrogen because of a history of breast cancer, uterine cancer, diabetes, vascular disorders, gallbladder disease, obesity, or a host of other problems for which estrogen was either totally or partially contraindicated. During these years our community had access to dual photon bone absorptiometry (DPA), a test that accurately measures bone mineral density. Osteoporosis could now be measured. I remembered that Dr. Peat had told of an over-the-counter cream (Cielo, it was called then) that contained good amounts of easily absorbed natural progesterone and was available at local health food stores. Since it had been used in cosmetics as a skin moisturizer for years and I found no references indicating any safety problems, I considered the progesterone cream safe to use.

So, in late 1979, I began recommending progesterone cream to my osteoporotic patients who could not use estrogen. Using annual serial DPA bone density tests, I followed the bone condition of these patients. To my considerable surprise, the bone mineral density tests showed that my patients using progesterone cream showed significant *increase* (average 15 percent) whereas my patients on estrogen alone showed no increase but either remained stable or actually *decreased*. In addition, the progesterone patients told me of one condition after another that had improved since they started using the cream. Their backaches had gone away, they slept better, they had more energy, they could lose weight more easily, their skin was less dry and less wrinkled, and their libido, which had more or less evaporated over the years, was now revived. And among those with a history of cancer, *none* had developed any recurrence or late metastases.

The increase in bone mineral density was particularly remarkable. In researching the medical literature, I could find no study reporting any similar results. Even the vaunted estrogen has never been found to increase bone mineral density; it only slows the bone loss of osteoporosis. And that meager benefit occurs only in the five- to six-year period around menopause time, after which osteoporosis bone loss continues at a rate of about 1.5 percent a year whether one takes estrogen or not. Fractures prevented, as advertised by the estrogen promoters, are actually only fractures delayed. It therefore seemed obvious to me to add natural progesterone cream to my patients already using estrogen. When I did, the same bone benefits appeared.

There was a problem, however. On adding progesterone, some of the patients complained of increased estrogen side effects such as water retention, fuller breasts, and weight gain. These all resolved when the estrogen dosage was reduced. This was my introduction into the mysteries of hormone balance. Each of these two important hormones increases the effect of the other. In nature's wisdom, the two hormones are meant to work together. Year after year, as I dealt with patient after patient, I learned more and more about the multiple ways in which these hormones affect the body. Things that once were mysterious became clear; things I thought I knew I discovered were more remarkable than I had dreamt. And, most wonderful of all, my treatment of hormonally related illnesses became based on understanding the underlying cause rather than on symptom-based prescriptions.

My library of books and papers on osteoporosis, breast cancer, menopause, uterine cancer, fibrocystic breasts, pregnancy, menarche, PMS, and hormones came to fill my shelves and accumulate in piles around my desk. In time, I wrote several papers on what I had observed in my patients. They found publication not in our U.S. mainstream journals (which demand placebo-controlled, double-blind studies), but in Australian, Canadian, English, and "alternative" journals. I talked to my colleagues and gave talks at our hospital staff meetings. The reception was warm but their looks of perplexity gave me to understand that I had hit what others have called "cognitive dissonance." While unable to dispute my work, my colleagues could not understand how the knowledge I presented was missing from their own education and the textbooks (and the pharmaceutical advertising) on which they relied. In their minds, the file marked "progesterone" was filled with advertising about synthetic progestins, which are not the same thing.

In 1993 I wrote a small book entitled *Natural Progesterone: The Multiple Roles of a Remarkable Hormone* in an attempt to explain to my colleagues everything I had learned about progesterone and women's hormone balance. Without any advertising, this little book has become a publishing success. In spite of its technical medical language, word has spread about this book and thousands of women, looking for the answers they haven't been getting anywhere else, have bought it. The informal networking among women on the subject of menopause and hormone balancing is a wonder to behold.

I teamed up with Virginia Hopkins to write this expanded and updated version of the book in lay language so that you would have easier access to information about the benefits of progesterone in a form that is straightforward, readable, and easy to use. We want you to know about the history and politics of the medical and drug establishment, to be extremely well informed about synthetic hormone replacement therapy, to understand the biochemistry and dynamics of your own hormones and how they get out of balance, and most of all, to learn how to prevent hormone imbalance and how to stay healthy. We have given you many guidelines for determining whether your hormones are out of balance as well as detailed information about how to use natural progesterone. We want to empower you to question your doctors intelligently; if you read this book from cover to cover, you are likely to be better informed on the subject of progesterone than they are. We hope that as you discover for yourself the truth of what is written here, you will insist that your doctor read it too, and continue the quiet but powerful revolution in knowledge and practice that is taking place regarding hormone replacement therapy.

There is a great thirst for knowledge in this field. Women know full well they are not being served properly by the treatments their doctors give them. They know something is wrong when 650,000 (or more) hysterectomies per year are performed in the United States. They know they are not victims of some mistake of Mother Nature. They know that a hormone that is supposed to cure them should not also promote cancer. Women are far more knowledgeable, intelligent, and intuitive than their doctors give them credit for. The word of progesterone's success has spread and a revolution in women's health care is under way.

But the full story of hormone replacement and hormone balancing has yet to be told. I'm sure that more discoveries and insights are ahead. Medicine is an ever-emerging science. With this book, I hope to add to the knowledge base that presently exists. It is a culmination of thirty-plus years of practice, fifteen years specifically studying progesterone, the reading of countless books and articles on the subject, and conversations with hundreds of doctors and thousands of women in my practice as well as the thousands of people who have contacted me to share their experiences since I wrote my earlier book, *Natural Progesterone*. This book will help women regain control of their own health destinies. When that happens, women will reeducate their doctors. It is my firm belief that our doctors need to be reeducated in the realities of their female patients' hormone matters. There is no teaching force for doctors more formidable or effective than knowledgeable, intelligent, assertive women. The book is dedicated to them.

This book would not have been possible without the expert assistance of my coauthor, science writer Virgina Hopkins. Her tireless dedication to the project, her communication and writing skills, and her attributes of applied women's wisdom have been indispensable not only to my understanding but to the understanding all readers will achieve concerning this important subject.

—John R. Lee, M.D.
Sebastopol, CA
June 1995

INTRODUCTION

The change. Every adult woman in North America and other industrialized countries knows what these words refer to: the "change of life" that occurs with menopause. Those who have entered into menopause know it by their own experience; others know the experience of their mothers, an older sister, or a friend. They have heard the stories of the hot flashes and night sweats, the mood swings, the vaginal dryness, and the sagging breasts and fatter hips. They vow (and pray) to somehow never let it happen that way to them. They fear the loss of sexual enjoyment that menopause may portend. They see older women shrunken and bent with osteoporosis, and cannot visit an older friend in a nursing home without some dread that this may be their destiny, too.

But they also know from other older women, who are vigorous and full of life, that this deterioration is not universal with all women. What, they wonder, makes the difference and what can be done to remain vital and healthy? Menopause, after all, is not a disease but only a transition between one's childbearing years and the large segment of life that follows when one no longer need be concerned with monthly menstrual bleeding and the possible responsibilities of pregnancy. Womanly intuition tells them that menopause is not a mistake of Mother Nature, a design error from which there is no escape. Women in other cultures appear to make this transition without all the problems we see here. Are they merely more stoic or do they have no audience for their complaints? Do they in fact sail through the change without any particular problem? Is there a difference and, if so, what makes it so?

Many menopause writers remind us that the general lack of medical history detailing menopausal changes in ages past can be explained by the shorter average life span common in earlier times. They point out that many mammals remain fertile throughout their lives and perhaps Mother Nature intended women to simply die when they were no longer able to carry children. This argument implies that our longer average life span is an unnatural extension of life created by our food abundance and improved medical care. Such reasoning is fallacious and should be put to rest.

Average life span does *not* mean that the average person died at such and such an age. It merely means that the age of death for a sufficiently large number of people born during a certain time period was recorded and used to calculate a numerical average. If, for example, during this time period half of the children died before age two and all the others lived to be eighty, the average life span would be about forty years. Or if no children died and everyone lived until forty and then died, their average life span would also be forty years. As it turns out, our longer life span is due almost solely to the decrease in childhood deaths from infectious diseases.

There were plenty of older women in European and American cultures during previous centuries. The average life span of our first seven presidents was longer than that of our most recently dead seven presidents. Saint Patrick, of Irish fame, is credited with living from 385 to 461 A.D. and this (76 years) was not thought to be particularly unusual at the time. Socrates was given poison hemlock to bring about his death in 399 B.C. when he was 70 years old. His contemporary, Plato, lived from 427 to 347 B.C. (80 years) and was not thought to be remarkably old. Though these examples are male, there is no time in history when women did not typically outlive males. I think we can safely discard the average life span argument as a basis for the lack of historical reports of menopause as a crisis in women's lives.

Others might argue that women's illnesses were not of sufficient importance to be included in medical writings of ages past. This, too, does not wash. Even though the typical doctor-historian was male, he would not refrain from writing about his success in treating such an important female malady if it existed.

Another argument I have heard is that the women's rights movement has used their media access to overstate the case regarding menopause problems. I have heard men exploit this argument to claim that U.S. women are spoiled. This also is nonsense, as anyone who treats these women can tell you. Any woman who goes through pregnancy and the delivery of a baby without undue complaint has got to be regarded as a strong and stoical person. When such a person tells me she is extremely distraught by uncontrollable hot flashes, night sweats, mood swings, depression, and the fear of osteoporosis, I tend to believe her.

The fact we must face is that women today are indeed suffering from a real menopausal disorder of which we have only a rudimentary understanding and for which our present mainstream treatments are simply not satisfactory. Our treatment with supplemental estrogen may reduce hot flashes and treat vaginal dryness, but it does so at the risk of inducing a higher incidence of endometrial cancer and breast cancer; it also causes unwanted fat and water retention. Consider the financial implications. Turning menopausal symptoms into a disease of estrogen deficiency has resulted in Premarin's being one of the top 10 prescription drugs sold in the United States. Let any American woman of menopausal age complain to her doctor of any symptom and the odds are she will receive a prescription for Premarin. Any symptom that persists after estrogen supplementation is considered trivial or cause for a tranquilizer prescription or a referral to a psychiatrist.

This symptom/drug approach points the way to what is amiss in mainstream medicine today. It suffers from a fixation on the drug treatment of health problems. The typical medical treatment program for almost any given health problem follows a war metaphor: Find the villain and destroy it. If a villain cannot be found, look for the destruction left in its wake. That is, treat the disease by killing it or, failing that, treat the symptoms. This was not the metaphor of conventional medicine of past centuries. Treatment concepts were previously directed at restoring balance in terms of physical, nutritional, emotional, environmental, and even spiritual factors.

Disease is often a late manifestation of a process that has its origin long before symptoms developed. This is certainly true of coronary heart disease, osteoporosis, breast and other cancers, fibroids, hypertension, arthritis, and many, many others. Mainstream medicine focuses on the disease as it becomes symptomatic, not on the initial asymptomatic stages. If we are to make any advance in health care, it will come as a result of understanding initial causes, not in waiting to treat the later symptomatic phase. A recent study in monkeys showed that diabetes and cardiovascular disease occurred rarely in monkeys that had been fed to remain slim, but almost exclusively in those monkeys allowed to get fat, even if they later had been put on a diet to lose their fat. Is this not a clue to guide us in the rearing of our own children?

Parallels abound throughout our present health care problems.

The majority of illnesses being treated today in the United States stems from preventable causes. A well-researched report in the 1993 issue of the *New England Journal of Medicine* states that *preventable illness makes up approximately 70 percent of the burden of disease and the associated costs.* By shifting our view from the mainstream disease-oriented categories to underlying causes, it is found that preventable causes account for eight of the nine leading categories and for 980,000 deaths per year.

We stand at the confluence of profound changes. Our present medical system is symptom-fixated and driven by misplaced economic incentives, but it now faces stiff competition from alternative practitioners. Women's health problems clustered under the banner of hormone balance are epidemic and not well addressed by mainstream medicine. Women are emerging from under a cloud of historic medical neglect and are rightly demanding new and more effective approaches. It is my hope that this book will provide guidance in this needed effort.

Since writing my book, *Natural Progesterone: The Multiple Roles of a Remarkable Hormone,* in 1993, I have had thousands of letters and phone calls from women describing the condescending, insensitive attitudes of their doctors in dealing (not very effectively) with their premenopause and menopause problems. A revolution is under way. Despite the lucrative incentives that sustain the present system, change will come because women demand it.

PART I

The Inner Workings of Hormone Balance

Chapter 1

THE CRUX OF THE MATTER: MENOPAUSAL POLITICS AND WOMEN'S HORMONE CYCLES

Not so long ago, *menopause* was a word you did not say out loud in public, and you had to go to a medical library to find a book on the subject. Go into a typical bookstore these days and you'll find literally dozens of titles on menopause. They range from praising the wonders of estrogen and hormone replacement therapy to personal stories of the ups and downs some women experience during the "change of life." What was once a taboo subject has become a mainstay of talk shows and women's magazine articles.

MENOPAUSAL POLITICS

With 30 million menopausal women in North America and some 20 million baby boomer women on the brink of menopause, it's no wonder this is a major topic of discussion. What *is* a wonder is how we have managed to make menopause, a perfectly natural part of a woman's life cycle, into a disease. It has only just dawned on us that menstruation, pregnancy, and childbirth are not diseases; now we need to realize that menopause is not a disease despite millions in advertising dollars spent by drug companies to convince us otherwise. The pharmaceutical companies have not failed to notice the huge population of premenopausal women in the pipeline, a financial gold mine in the making. Premarin, a form of hormone replacement therapy made from pregnant mare's urine by the Wyeth-Ayerst Company, is already one of the top-selling prescription medicines in the United States. And so far they've only managed to capture 10 to 15 percent of the market! Industry projections of hormone replacement sales overall by the year 2000 are up to a billion dollars a year! Estimates put Premarin's 1992 sales worldwide at nearly $700 million, and in 1994, Premarin ranked as number 8 in dollar volume in pharmaceutical products, up 12 percent from 1993. A large percentage of advertising and research dollars are spent trying to convince women that estrogen will cure everything from heart disease to Alzheimer's, but there is scant evidence for any of these claims and reams of evidence that synthetic estrogens are highly toxic and carcinogenic.

The good news is that women have become guarded and skeptical about having new drugs pushed on them. After being told that DES, a hormone that was supposed to guard against miscarriages, was safe, hundreds of thousands of women discovered the hard way that it caused cancer in their children. Women were told that Valium was a safe and effective remedy for depression, only to find out that it was addictive. Now their physicians are trying to convince them that once they have reached menopause they should automatically go on hormone replacement therapy featuring synthetic estrogens and progestins. So far, only 10 to 15 percent of menopausal women have chosen to follow this advice despite intense pressure on all women from their doctors and the media. The real tragedy is that the natural forms of these hormones, used wisely and in moderation, could be of very real benefit to millions of women. I believe that the present synthetic versions of hormones are making millions of women sick and putting them at risk for cancer, strokes, and heart disease. In the chapters that follow, we will look more closely at how estrogen and progesterone work in a woman's body and the politics of pushing drugs to women.

WHAT IS MENOPAUSE?

Strictly speaking, menopause is the cessation of menses, the end of menstrual cycles. The unpleasant "symptoms" of menopause that some women suffer, such as hot flashes, vaginal dryness, and mood swings, are peculiar to Western industrialized cultures and, as far as I can tell, they are virtually unknown in the Far East and third-world countries. In native cultures menopause tends to be a cause for quiet celebration, a time when a woman has completed her childbearing years and is moving into a deeper level of self-discovery and spiritual awareness. She is becoming a wise old woman. In these cultures menopausal women are looked up to and revered. They are sought out for advice and their opinions are heavily weighed in the decision-making process of the community. How strange that sounds to us! We know menopause as a death knell, the end of a woman's sexuality, a descent into a dried-up and painful old age of arthritis and osteoporosis. How did this experience of menopause come to be? I believe it's a combination of poor diet, unhealthy lifestyle, environmental pollutants, cultural attitudes, the incorrect use of synthetic hormones, and advertising. But first, let's look at what happens in a woman's body as menopause approaches.

THE RISE AND FALL OF HORMONES DURING THE MENSTRUAL CYCLE

In a normal menstrual cycle, every 26 to 28 days the ovaries, which hold a woman's eggs, receive a hormonal signal from the brain that it's time to get some eggs ready to be fertilized. Anywhere from a few to a few hundred eggs begin to mature inside sacs called follicles. After 10 to 12 days one egg has moved to the outer surface of the ovary and the follicle bursts, releasing the egg into the fallopian tube for its journey to the uterus. The follicle then becomes the corpus luteum.

As the egg is ripening in the ovary, the uterus is ripening in preparation for the possibility of growing a fetus. The uterine lining thickens and becomes engorged with blood that will nourish the growing embryo. If no fertilized egg implants itself in the uterus, it sheds its lining. This shedding is the blood of menstruation. Then the cycle begins again, with the signal from the brain telling the ovary to ripen an egg.

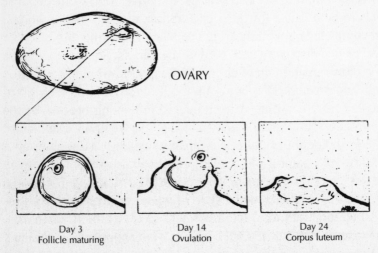

OVARY

| Day 3 | Day 14 | Day 24 |
| Follicle maturing | Ovulation | Corpus luteum |

Figure 1: Ovulation of a follicle

Estrogen (from *estrus*, meaning "heat" or "fertility") is the dominant hormone for the first week or so after menstruation, stimulating the buildup of tissue and blood in the uterus as the ovarian follicles simultaneously begin their development of the egg. Around the time of ovulation, estrogen causes changes in the vaginal mucus, making it more tolerant of male penetration during sexual activity and more hospitable to sperm. At this phase in the menstrual cycle, the vaginal mucus tends to somewhat resemble uncooked egg whites. Watching for this change in mucus combined with a rise in body temperature is one of the best non-laboratory methods for identifying the time of ovulation.

About twelve days after the beginning of the previous menstruation, the rising estrogen level peaks and then tapers off just as the follicle matures and just before ovulation. After ovulation the now-empty follicle becomes the corpus luteum (so named because of its appearance as a small yellow body on the surface of the ovary). The corpus luteum is the site of progesterone production, which dominates the second half of the menstrual month, reaching a peak of about 20 milligrams per day.

Progesterone production during this phase of the cycle, along with estrogen, leads to a refinement and "ripening" of tissue and blood in the uterus. Progesterone also contributes to the changes in the vaginal mucus seen at the time of ovulation. The rise of progesterone at the time of ovulation causes a rise of body temperature of about one degree Fahrenheit, a finding often used to indicate ovulation.

If pregnancy does not occur within 10 to 12 days after ovulation, estrogen and progesterone levels fall abruptly, triggering menstruation, and the cycle begins anew. If pregnancy occurs, progesterone production increases and the shedding of the lining of the uterus is prevented, thus preserving the developing embryo. As pregnancy progresses, progesterone production is taken over by the placenta and its secretion increases gradually to levels of 300 to 400 milligrams per day during the third trimester.

PREMENOPAUSE

A woman's hormone balance can begin to shift at anywhere from her midthirties to her late forties, depending on a variety of factors such as heredity, environment, how early or late she began menstruating, whether she had children and if so at what age and how many, and her lifestyle. Was she exhausted trying to juggle career and family? Was she eating junk food, caffeine, sugar, and alcohol or whole grains, fresh vegetables, and fruits? Has she taken vitamins? Has she lived in the city or country? Was she exposed to toxins in the workplace? Hormone balance is intimately connected to stress levels, nutrition, and the environmental toxins encountered daily. We will discuss all of these factors more thoroughly in the chapters to come.

The ability of the follicles to mature an egg and release it may begin "sputtering," so to speak, a decade before actual menopause, creating menstrual cycles in which a woman does not ovulate, called *anovulatory* cycles. If she isn't ovulating, she isn't producing progesterone from the ovaries and she may begin experiencing menopausal symptoms such as weight gain, water retention, and mood swings. Menstrual cycles can continue even without the progesterone, however, so most women aren't aware that the lack of progesterone is causing their symptoms. This is known as perimenopause, or premenopause. We will be discussing what I call "premenopause syndrome" in detail in Chapter 11.

It used to be true that the majority of women began menopause in their midforties to early fifties. In the last generation, however, things appear to have changed. Women now may have anovulatory periods starting in their early thirties and yet do not experience cessation of periods (menopause) until their fifties. During this time, the ovaries continue to produce estrogen sufficient for regular or irregular shedding, creating what I term "estrogen dominance," which will be discussed in detail throughout the book. Some women may go for years with irregular cycles and slowly wind down, or may just suddenly stop menstruating one month and never menstruate again. They may be overwhelmed with unpleasant symptoms or hardly notice what has happened other than not having to worry about birth control or buy tampons every month. How menopause is experienced is as individual and unique as each human being.

During the many months of anovulatory periods, estrogen production may become erratic, with surges of inappropriately high levels alternating with irregular low levels. Periods of vaginal bleeding may become erratic, some much heavier than others. When estrogen surges, women undergoing these changes may notice breast swelling and tenderness, mood swings, sleep disturbance, water retention, and a tendency to put on weight. These may be the symptoms of estrogen dominance caused mainly by lack of ovulation and thereby lack of progesterone while their estrogen levels are still in the "normal" range. Their doctors may check their estradiol levels and their FSH and LH levels, but rarely does it dawn on them that their patients' progesterone levels are too low. In taking the usual blood tests, the doctor may find the estrogen normal that day or even a bit on the low side and FSH levels a bit too high. On another day the estrogen might be elevated and FSH levels normal. If the former is found, the doctor may even prescribe some estrogen on the theory that the patient is nearing true menopause. The woman usually finds that this does not help her.

More often, the doctor ascribes her complaints to emotional causes or simply some defect of Mother Nature that women must endure. In later chapters, I will discuss this phenomenon in more detail. For the present, we will merely say that a rising percentage of women are experiencing premenopausal woes that are related to their hormones. The details concerning environmental toxins, nutritional factors, stress, adrenal hormones, exercise, and weight will be found in the chapters ahead.

Chapter 2

THE DANCE OF THE STEROIDS

The word *steroids* may conjure up visions of muscle-bound body-builders and unpleasant side effects, but steroid is really a generic name for dozens of body regulators (hormones) made from cho-le*sterol*. Cholesterol, the basic building block for the steroid hormones, gives them all a similar structure. An analogy would be a basic clothing ensemble. You begin with a beige jacket and matching slacks. Add a blouse, a necklace, and some pumps and you have a business outfit for a corporate office. Or add a scoop neck silk blouse, cut the jacket at the waist, and you're ready for a night on the town. Or make the jacket and slacks a darker color, add a button-down shirt, some epaulets and gold braid, and you have a military uniform. The basic suit stays the same but the additions, subtractions, and other alterations make the difference in the role you play. In the same sense, all the steroid molecules resemble cholesterol in their basic structure. Switch a few atoms around and the role of the hormone can change dramatically.

Without sufficient cholesterol, we can't make sufficient steroid hormones. (If you would like to see how biochemists picture the cholesterol molecule, turn to the appendix on page 356.) Some of the other more familiar steroids are estrogen, progesterone, testosterone, the corticosteroids, and DHEA. The steroid drugs that bodybuilders use are called anabolic steroids. Anabolic means that they have a "building" function rather than a "taking apart" function. Testosterone, for example, helps build up muscle mass, as do some corticosteroids. Although the workings of the steroids are subtle and complex, a slight imbalance can have major effects. Learning a bit about steroid hormones can give you an enormous advantage in making informed decisions about hormone replacement therapy. What I am about to tell you here, most doctors forgot a long time ago, but the information is fundamental to truly understanding hormone balance.

The first step in the body's manufacture of steroid hormones from cholesterol happens in tiny energy packets called mitochondria found within every cell of the body except red blood cells. From cholesterol, the mitochondria make a hormone called pregnenolone, which, as it passes through the bloodstream to the ovaries and adrenal glands, can then be transformed into progesterone or (almost identical) 17-OH-pregnenolone. Then, from these two steroids, progesterone and 17-OH-pregnenolone, all the other steroid hormones can be made by relatively minor molecular modifications, depending on body need. In this sort of production, one steroid is transformed into another. Many of the steps along the steroid pathway are active hormones in their own right even though they also serve by being transformed into yet other hormones (see Figure 2).

Although the steroid hormones are remarkably similar in shape, each of them has markedly different effects, and these differences arise from very slight variations in their molecular structure. Let's look at some of the major players in this constantly shifting milieu of steroid hormones.

THE CAST OF MAJOR PLAYERS

Pregnenolone—Synthesized from cholesterol by mitochondria of all the cells of the body (except red blood cells), this molecule is the precursor to all steroid hormones.

Progesterone—A precursor to most of the steroid hormones, it is responsible for a myriad of important jobs from maintaining pregnancy to regulating menstrual cycles. Made primarily in the ovaries, it is described in detail in later chapters.

17α-OH-progesterone—A variant of progesterone, it leads to cortisol production in the adrenal cortex and to androstenedione from which all other sex hormones are made.

DHEA (dehydroepiandrosterone)—A precursor to the androgens, testosterone, and the estrogens, DHEA is important to protein building and repair. Most likely it has other important jobs as well that are still being discovered. It is made primarily in the adrenal glands. DHEA levels decline dramatically as we age, making it a primary biomarker of aging.

Androstenedione and Androstenediol—Androgenic (masculinizing) hormones, they are precursors to testosterone and the estrogens. Produced in the ovaries and the adrenals from either progesterone or DHEA, they are the source of estrogen production after menopause or loss of one's ovaries.

17-OH-pregnenolone—A modification of pregnenolone created in the adrenal cortex, testes, and ovarian follicles, it is used in the adrenal cortex and testes to create DHEA. In the ovaries it is an alternate step for 17∝-OH-progesterone production.

Testosterone—A male sex hormone that stimulates the growth of male characteristics and the production of sperm, it is a precursor to the estrogens. It is made primarily in the testes but also in much smaller amounts by the ovaries.

Estrone, Estradiol, and Estriol—Female sex hormones known as estrogen, they are primarily responsible for the growth of female characteristics in puberty and regulating the menstrual cycle. They are made primarily in the ovaries but also from androstenedione in fat cells, muscle cells, and skin even after menopause.

Corticosterone, Cortisol—They help regulate numerous bodily functions including glucose and energy balance; they also moderate inflammation and immune responses throughout the body. They are made in the adrenal glands.

Aldosterone—Made in the adrenal glands, it controls sodium and potassium levels in the blood and is important in regulating electrolytes and blood pressure.

Their position in the biosynthesis pathway is indicated by the following diagram:

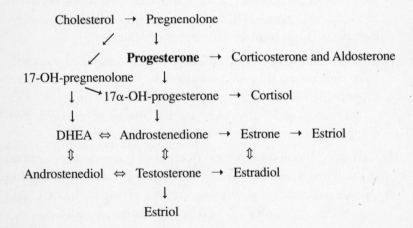

Figure 2: Basic steroid hormone pathways in the ovary, testis, and adrenal gland. Each arrow in the pathway diagram represents the work of a specific enzyme. The arrow symbol was chosen because it indicates the direction of the action. Only in a few instances is an action reversible, as indicated by the double arrows.

CHOREOGRAPHING THE DANCE

The steroid hormones shown in the diagram above are made primarily in the ovaries of women, the testes of men, and the adrenal glands of both sexes. As far as we know, all of the steroid hormones are made from cholesterol. This is one of the reasons it is so important *not* to go on a no-fat or no-cholesterol diet. Although our body can manufacture about 75 percent of our cholesterol from other foods we eat, the remaining 25 percent comes directly from cholesterol-containing foods. Eliminate cholesterol entirely and hormone imbalance may be the result. Low cholesterol in the elderly has been linked to depression and suicide. As in most things, moderation and balance are the answer. The transformation from one hormone to another requires an enzyme, which in turn require vitamin and mineral *cofactors*. A substance that is the source of another substance is called the *precursor*. (If you would like more detailed biochemical information about the enzymes in the steroid pathways, please see the appendix on page 356.)

THE JOURNEY ALONG THE STEROID HORMONE PATHWAY

As I describe the pathways in words, follow my description on the diagram on page 14 (Figure 2).

The journey begins on the upper left corner with pregnenolone having been derived from cholesterol. The flow of hormones then progresses from pregnenolone along one of two major pathways: one to the left and down through the adrenal DHEA (dehydroepiandrosterone) pathway, or straight down through progesterone in both the ovarian and adrenal glands. Both pathways lead to what we call metabolic end points. Aldosterone, cortisol, and the estrogens are the final stops, or metabolic end points, on the steroid hormone pathways.

With the exception of the end point hormones, all of the steroid hormone molecules are capable of being converted into some other molecule. Testosterone, for instance, can be a precursor of the estrogen called estradiol, and androstenedione can be a precursor of either testosterone or estrone, another estrogen. Estrone and estradiol can be interchanged into each other via a redox (reduction/oxidation) system in the liver. Progesterone is a precursor in several pathways, one leading to androstenedione and on to the estrogens and to testosterone, another to cortisol, and another to corticosterone and aldosterone. Similarly, DHEA is a precursor in the pathway leading to testosterone and androstenedione, the latter leading on to the estrogens but *not* to other corticosteroids.

The ebb and flow of steroid hormones along their pathways is a result of enzyme action monitored and controlled by biofeedback mechanisms evolved over eons of time in the limbic brain (hypothalamus). It is important to realize that enzyme (and hormone) function is dependent on precise molecular configuration. Enzymes are large molecules continuously created from blueprints in our chromosomes, which generally require specific vitamin and mineral cofactors to maximize their job of transforming one hormone into another. (That is why a healthy diet and vitamin/mineral supplements can be so effective in helping your body work right.) Each enzyme performs but one function, such as the splitting of a single chemical bond in a specific molecule. To perform that one function, an enzyme must precisely "fit" the structure of the molecule, like a complicated key-and-lock system. Molecular conformation, or the exact and specific structure of the molecules, is the key to the smooth running of these enzyme pathways.

Molecular conformation is the factor that distinguishes natural hormones most strongly from the synthetic versions sold by drug companies. Synthetic hormones have altered shapes not known in nature, created by the addition of atoms at unusual positions. Thus, synthetic steroids, such as those found in the typical hormone replacement therapy (HRT) prescription, are not subject to the usual enzymatic pathways. We don't naturally have enzymes designed to handle any of the synthetic steroids; their effects cannot be "tuned down" or "turned off" as needed, nor can they be efficiently excreted through the usual enzymatic mechanisms. Despite their advertisements, synthetic hormones are not equivalent to natural hormones. Harmony and balance, the hallmark of a healthy body, are lost when biologically active synthetic compounds are thrown into the dance of the steroids. The mischief they can create in the normal ebb and flow of vital steroid hormones is most likely responsible for a great deal of hormonal imbalance.

THE DANCE OF THE STEROIDS

Understanding steroids requires a vision into the unseen. Humans have the power to create reality beyond their normal experience. We do it all the time with music, books, stories, fantasies, dreams, and, yes, especially in science. Science is really the art of "seeing" forces and elements invisible to the normal senses. No physicist has ever seen an atom, yet she conjures an image to understand them. We know that atoms join together to create molecules. Although the atomic bonding necessary to create molecules involves a sharing of electrons not well understood, we can still glean information from nature's hidden forces. We can learn to understand, to use, and even to create molecules. In the "movements" that follow, I will describe my vision of the world of the biological molecules we call steroid hormones, based on my understanding of biochemistry. I call this vision "the dance of the steroids." Think of it as action accompanied by music. Do not try to understand this vision with your logical, linear mind; allow your intuitive mind to grasp it for you.

FOUR MOVEMENTS:
THE FLOW OF STEROIDS IN OUR BODIES

Movement 1. Andante con molto

There is a land near but far away where busy workers by the millions are doing the work of the body in beautiful, flowing, complex harmony. These are the steroids, turning out products to match our needs, stabilizing, energizing, and nurturing our cells and tissues; ensuring repair and replication of vital body parts; protecting us against damage; and, for a great portion of our adult life, fostering the genesis and development of a new life to carry on the species after our own body ceases to exist. The landscape is alive with hustle and bustle but the prevailing mode is one of synchrony and balance, busy but harmonious. Life is throbbing in a ceaseless flow of energy. We sense the magnitude of activity, the surgings and ebbings of rhythms unseen, and the ungraspable complexity of it all. But at the same time we are aware of order, coordination, and purpose. Despite the complexity and energy apparent, there is an air of majesty and design.

Movement 2. Adagio

A collection of still photographs reveals workers at their benches, bakers busy in their shops, potters at their kilns, carpenters at their labor, homemakers in their nests, firemen at their stations, police standing vigilant, nurses doing their tending, and a host of activities beyond our understanding. At first glance, the workers all look identical. Closer examination reveals slight differences among the various classes of workers. They all seem to be made of the same parts but with minor variations in how the parts are put together. We see that without exception the minor differences among the workers strictly correlate with the work each is doing. Though all are steroids, each is designed with a specific job in mind. What at first appeared to us as chaos is only a fault in our understanding. Precision and synchrony are paramount.

Movement 3. Allegro con brio

Live video captures the hustle and bustle of myriad activities, the arrival of raw materials and the departure of finished products, and the ceaseless inflow of new workers and the outflow of workers apparently called elsewhere. Just off camera, we are told, are the cholesterol molecules having their parts rearranged to enter the scene as worker units. To our amazement, some workers will, in the blink of an eye, be suddenly transformed from baker to chef, from nurse to fireman, from carpenter to potter, without a hint of discontinuity or a missed beat in their activities. Their parts will have been suddenly rearranged and their functions switched simultaneously with their newly acquired form. This magical transformation is accomplished by shimmering protein globules (enzymes) passing amongst them, briefly embracing each selected worker molecule and, in a flash of electromagnetic energy, leaving them with slightly altered elements and new functions, impressing upon the whole scene a synchrony of design and purpose.

Movement 4. Largo maestoso

Some of the molecules, having reached an end point in their transformational process, are kept in balanced concentration by being gently swept along in an invisible current to distant parts (the liver) where, their work being done, they are wedded (conjugated) to bile acids and carried silently off our viewing screen. Scientists would say that they are inactivated by hydroxylation (in the case of estrogens) or hydrogenated and conjugated with glucuronic acid (in the case of progesterone) for excretion in bile. On the periphery of our video scene is a continuous magical influx of new worker units sufficient to meet the rise and fall of their essential functions. In this manner, excesses and/or deficiencies are well prevented and a sense of order pervades.

Now that your intuitive mind has had some fun, you can go back to your logical, linear mind. For those interested in the whole tableau of the biosynthetic pathways complete with their molecular structure, the known enzymes (and their vitamin and mineral cofactors) that perform the transformation, and the gland tissue(s) in which each step takes place, turn to the appendix on page 356. You will be able to follow the transformations by simply following the arrows. It is time now to get on with a look at the history of hormone replacement.

Chapter 3

THE HISTORY OF HORMONE REPLACEMENT THERAPY AND THE ESTROGEN MYTH

Estrogen replacement therapy (ERT) was first conceived in the late 1950s, the era of "better living through chemistry." These were the heady, innocent postwar years when enthusiasm for controlling the natural environment with chemicals was matched only by the eagerness of the chemical companies to find a profitable use for their products. Concurrently, pharmaceutical companies were discovering the financial gains to be made by a similar philosophy: For every human ailment there is a drug that will cure it. Pesticides and antibiotics were going to save the human race.

Both the chemical and pharmaceutical companies were learning the value of cleverly disguised public relations campaigns in which articles extolling the virtues of a product were "planted" in magazines and newspapers. The media went along with this approach (and still do), reaping huge benefits in advertising dollars from these same companies. The public naïvely believed (and still do) that if they read it in a major publication, it must be true. Few industries have reaped more benefits from this public naïveté than pharmaceutical companies. The practice continues unabated to this day; the major women's magazines are a virtual pipeline of information for drug companies eager to push their products under the guise of editorial neutrality.

The burgeoning awareness in American industry that the media could be easily manipulated to push their products took place in a cultural milieu that placed an emphasis on the nuclear family, with the father out earning a living and the mother at home with a baby on her hip and a batch of cookies in the oven. The ultra-feminine Marilyn Monroe was the cultural ideal of beauty. Women were thought to be at their best pleasing their husbands sexually and raising healthy, happy children. It's no coincidence that ERT was born just as the first big wave of American women raised to be happy homemakers was approaching middle age and menopause. Their children were leaving home, their hair was turning gray, and their breasts were sagging. Symbolically, their usefulness had come to an end: If they were no longer raising children, and no longer sexually attractive to their husbands, of what use were they? Psychological problems such as depression became common among women of this age. Millions of women became hooked on "mother's little helpers," Valium and other tranquilizers.

MENOPAUSE BECOMES A DISEASE

Meanwhile, Ayerst, the first maker of a conjugated estrogen called Premarin, found the goose that laid the golden public relations egg in a Brooklyn, New York, gynecologist named Dr. Robert A. Wilson. With a list of sterling credentials as long as his arm, a dash of charisma, a zeal for keeping women young and feminine, and plenty of money from the pharmaceutical industry, Wilson hit the streets with the good news about estrogen. He used adjectives bordering on lurid to describe menopause deprecatingly as a time when women became dried-up, cranky, sexless old hags. His magic pill was going to save them from that "tragedy," keeping them "feminine forever." To make matters worse, it seems that almost everyone researching or writing about menopause from that point on quoted Wilson and unquestioningly accepted his information as fact, when in fact most of it was fiction.

If one were to pick a year during which ERT entered public consciousness, it might be 1964. The January 13, 1964, issue of *Newsweek* carried a one-page story entitled "No More Menopause?" reporting on the work of Dr. Wilson, who was reported to have been studying menopause since the 1920s. He had reached the conclusion that "change of life" stemmed from a lack of the female hormones estrogen and progesterone.

Meanwhile, an enterprising and unhappily menopausal writer in London named Ann Walsh happened to read the *Newsweek* article with great interest. She was immediately struck by the great similarity between Wilson's description of what happens when one's ovaries stop functioning and her own disturbing set of symptoms. Walsh returned to the United States for a whirlwind tour of interviews with as many medical authorities involved in hormone research as she could track down. Their consistently cautionary tone about estrogen did not dampen her enthusiasm in the least. By late 1965 she produced a book titled *Now! The Pills to Keep Women Young! ERT The First Complete Account of the Miracle Hormone Treatment That May Revolutionize the Lives of Millions of Women!* Shortly thereafter, Dr. Wilson produced his own book entitled *Feminine Forever,* copies of which were quickly disseminated to doctors' offices by Ayerst detail men (sales reps for pharmaceutical firms) throughout the United States, including my own office in Mill Valley, California.

In the years of 1964 and 1965, the lay press suddenly blossomed with ERT articles. Following the January 1964 *Newsweek* article, there appeared the following:

Pageant (August 1964) "No More Menopause"

Ladies' Home Journal (January 1965) "The Truth About Female Hormones"

Good Housekeeping (April 1965) "Menopause: Is It Necessary?"

Time (April 16, 1965) "The Springs of Youth"

Cosmopolitan (July 1965) "Oh, What a Lovely Pill"

Vogue (August 15, 1965) "How to Live Young at Any Age— Straight Talk About Hormones from a Famous Doctor"

McCall's (October 1965) "E.R.T.: Pills to Keep You Young" (by Ann Walsh herself)

The economic impact of the ERT revolution was not lost on the financially minded: even the *Wall Street Journal* carried a couple of lead articles on the subject. What woman wouldn't want to maintain her youth and femininity forever?

THE TRUTH BEHIND THE HOOPLA

In truth, estrogen had been very poorly researched. Its approval as a prescription drug was based on a dubious study with a relatively small number of women in Puerto Rico who took birth control pills. The pill used at first was only a progestin, which was later found to be contaminated with estrogen-like substances. When estrogen was taken out of the birth control pills, they didn't work as well, so a synthetic estrogen was intentionally added.

Twenty percent of the women in the study complained of side effects, but they were dismissed as neurotic. The three women who died while taking these pills were not autopsied to find out the cause of death. There has been ample evidence since then that these pills caused blood clots and strokes, but that evidence was dismissed and suppressed for the supposedly higher good of controlling the population explosion. Meanwhile, the pharmaceutical companies scrambled to find a combination of synthetic hormones that had fewer side effects. As Paula B. Doress-Worters said in a foreword to Sandra Coney's excellent book, *The Menopause Industry: How the Medical Establishment Exploits Women*:

> Hormone therapy has been called a product in search of a market. Most research on menopause is designed to demonstrate the desirability of medicalized interventions. Although the use of hormones to help women cope with common signs of menopause, such as hot flashes, has been known since 1937, hormone treatment was popularized for a mass market in the 1960s. It was promoted not simply as a palliative for the discomforts of menopause but also as a panacea for "psychological problems" supposedly related to the change of life. Such claims were unproven but were treated as common knowledge. These assertions promoted a stereotyped view of postmenopausal older women as asexual, neurotic, and unattractive. As a result, exogenous estrogen was approved for prescription use without adequate testing and soon became one of the five top-selling prescription drugs.

From 1965 to the mid-1970s, the ERT bandwagon sailed along with more and more women opting for the little pills that would keep them young. By 1975, however, a dark cloud emerged: Women on ERT were developing uterine (endometrial) cancer at a rate four to eight times greater than in untreated women. Multiple researchers confirmed the link between estrogen supplementation and uterine (endometrial) cancer. When the bad news hit

the newspapers, sales of estrogen supplements dropped precipi-
tously. Not only were women deciding not to start ERT and those
on ERT deciding to quit, but physicians were understandably re-
luctant to prescribe it, despite its apparent virtues.

But the estrogen bandwagon was only temporarily stalled.
After a spate of papers arguing the question of whether estrogen
"caused" endometrial cancer or merely "promoted" it (a distinc-
tion lost on most female patients and their doctors), medical authorities pulled themselves together and switched from ERT to
HRT (hormone replacement therapy).

The difference was the addition of the progestins (synthetic
versions of progesterone). Fairly solid research existed or was
soon accomplished to show that only "unopposed" estrogen was
the culprit; estrogen combined with progestins actually prevented
endometrial cancer. Endometrial cancer was unknown in women
whose ovaries produced a proper balance of estrogen and progesterone. Research by Dr. R. Don Gambrell, Jr., of the Medical College of Georgia and also by Dr. Lila E. Nachtigall at the
Goldwater Memorial Hospital in New York City revealed that, in
women on a combined treatment program of estrogen with progestin the incidence of uterine cancer was considerably less than
in controls (women not receiving hormones).

The parallel fear of estrogen causing breast cancer was addressed in the same manner. Studies of women on HRT were reported to show less breast cancer than in women not on HRT.
Whether this question was truly resolved or not, the ERT bandwagon was soon back on track as the HRT bandwagon.

The promoters of HRT also decided that estrogen and progestins could cure other ills, and were soon declaring that HRT would
also lower a woman's risk of heart disease and prevent osteoporosis. These assertions were followed by massive marketing
campaigns to "popularize" osteoporosis and educate women
about it. I have had literally hundreds of women tell me that their

doctors have "threatened" them ominously with predictions of heart disease and osteoporosis if they didn't take estrogen—regardless of whether they had any risk whatsoever for these diseases! The first assertion, that estrogen protects women from heart disease, is very debatable, as you will read in more detail in Chapter 13, and the second, that it reverses osteoporosis, is blatantly untrue, but these myths persist. Most people don't have the medical background to check and question the original research from which these assertions are made.

Somewhere early in the development of the HRT industry, progesterone was not only forgotten, it was mislabeled and mistaken as its distant cousins, the synthetic progestins. Even well-researched books on menopause tend to make this error: They never question whether the use of natural hormones might have some benefit, and they never question what happened to natural progesterone.

In rereading the early papers on estrogen replacement therapy I can sense the zeal and honest conviction of the authors. However, in retrospect, I can also see the narrowness of their views. They failed to ask some important questions, such as: Do women in other cultures experience the same menopausal symptoms and, if not, why not? Are there other causal factors operating here? What about side effects such as weight gain, water retention, migraine headaches, breast swelling, and fibrocystic breasts? Why do symptoms start before menopause, when estrogen levels are still high? Whatever happened to progesterone? What about HRT side effects of progestins? Within a specific culture, are symptom differences among women related to exercise, diet, or work environment? Their enthusiasm for estrogen seemed to blind them to this wider view.

It has been assumed that most women suffer from menopause symptoms. However, in checking the research, I can find no solid evidence to back up this assumption; most of it is anecdotal. My own hunch, based on 30 years of family practice and conversations with thousands of women around the country, is that a small percentage of women suffer from severe enough hot flashes and vaginal dryness to warrant treatment with natural hormones. Then there is a large population of women in their midthirties and on up suffering from the symptoms of estrogen dominance brought on by a sedentary lifestyle, a poor diet, birth control pills, HRT, and exposure to environmental estrogens. Many of these women can find relief simply through exercise and a good diet. Others can solve their problems with a few herbs, vitamins, and mineral supplements. Most of the rest find relief by using a natural progesterone cream. My observation is that estrogen is only needed by a very small percentage of women, and then only for a short time.

Sandra Coney, author of *The Menopause Industry,* carefully researched the claims made about how ill menopausal women really are. She has also found *no* good evidence that the majority of menopausal women are unhealthy, suffer debilitating symptoms, or lose their sex drive. Those women showing up in doctors' offices with problems are the ones who have had their uterus and/or ovaries removed, a very specific kind of menopause. Menopause as a disease has been largely fabricated by physicians and the pharmaceutical industry. Moreover, there is also no evidence to support the claims that estrogen retards aging, keeping women "young and feminine" forever. On the contrary, for most women it has unpleasant side effects ranging from annoying to life-threatening.

PERPETUATING THE ESTROGEN MYTH

Given the above, one might ask: How does this estrogen-deficiency mindset maintain its hold on the medical profession and the public? Is there some sort of censorship that controls what is published in our journals? The answer is yes and no. There is no formal censorship, but there is an economic incentive that subtly persaudes the policies of advertisement-dominated journals to continue the estrogen myth. Consider the following by Jerilynn C. Prior, M.D., an endocrinology professor at the University of British Columbia, Vancouver, British Columbia, excerpted from an article she wrote entitled "One Voice on Menopause." Her words speak for themselves:

He spoke carefully, choosing his words, "Maybe you had better not write it, then. I'd hate to see you put effort into it and then be unable to have it published."

I had been invited to be an author for a short, practical chapter on osteoporosis for a monograph for family doctors about menopause treatment. I was telephoning the editor, a young academic gynecologist, to ask for guidelines about my chapter. As we talked, it became clear what I was expected to write: *All menopausal women need estrogen treatment to prevent osteoporosis.*

"Thank you anyway," he said. "Good-bye."

As I hung up the phone I felt a great mixture of feelings. At first I was relieved. I can certainly manage without an additional deadline! Then I was filled with a bitter chagrin—I was dismissed and neatly eliminated from the scene. I was not allowed to say what I thought was true and what I felt would be helpful for doctors and their patients. The worldview of this gynecologist left no place for honest scientific debate. When all those feelings had settled, I was angry. How dare he impose his view of the world on me and, for that matter, on women! With no hesitation, he had defined a natural phase of life, inevitable for half the world's population, as a disease.

I am the first to admit that I am not a menopause expert. I am only a perimenopausal woman with 15 years of practice in reproductive endocrinology who has conducted (and been able to publish a few) prospective studies of reproduction. My own ex-

periences, the histories of my patients, and the science that is
pertinent, prospective, and randomized leave me deeply skeptical that menopause is a medical liability and, most of all, that estrogen deficiency is the major problem. I am astonished, for
example, at how little "science" prepared me for my own perimenopausal experiences. The current view that estrogen levels
gradually decrease in cycles that become longer and then scant
before the last flow is based on a study of eight selected women
who had blood drawn daily across one cycle that was some un-
specified duration into the four years of the usual menopause
transition. In contrast to this, in the last two years I have had hot
flashes and night sweats and I haven't missed one menstrual period. I continue to have cycles that are normal or short in interval, tend to be heavy in flow, and, with two exceptions, have
been absolutely normal in ovulatory characteristics (normal
luteal phase length of ten or more days).

What if I had told this editor that I believe I am currently experiencing estrogen excess? Otherwise, I find it hard to explain my
short follicular phases, early and increased cervical mucus production, short cycles, breast enlargement, and nipple tenderness. Is
my experience a figment of my imagination? What I have learned
from my own experience, has, however, been reported. . . .

Neugarten, for example, found that the symptoms of perimenopausal women resembled those of adolescents more than
those of postmenopausal women (with the exception that adolescents had fewer hot flushes). When breast tenderness, weight
gain, bloating, and mood changes occur in adolescence, however, they are ascribed to high estrogen exposure. Yet, when
these same symptoms are experienced during the transition to
menopause, they are caused by "estrogen deficiency!"

I flashed back to my telephone conversation. He was not
pleased when I said I thought menopause was a normal phase of
every woman's life. No, it would be too confusing to write that.
"The literature clearly indicates that menopause causes heart disease and osteoporosis. Also, it causes vasomotor symptoms,

mood changes, decreased sex drive, and other problems," he said. I said I would write that each woman herself must make the final decision about whether or not to take hormone treatment. He responded glibly, "Of course, but doctors must tell each woman that she is estrogen deficient so she will make the right choice."

"How would you feel if you knew you were condemned to become diseased when you reached your late forties or early fifties?" I said.

He didn't answer. Instead he retorted, "If I were a woman, I would take estrogen."

"But some women don't feel well on estrogen," I protested.

"Estrogen treatment, I mean hormone treatment," he corrected himself, knowing my belief that progesterone is also an important female hormone, "is benign. Most women tolerate hormone treatment very well."

When I didn't answer, he went on, "I have colleagues coming from all over asking me to put their 40-year-old wives on estrogen so they won't get heart attacks."

"Why aren't the 40-year-old wives *themselves* coming?" I asked gently, now feeling helpless.

He didn't answer my question.

Perhaps, I thought to myself, those 40-year-old wives of physicians didn't feel diseased. Maybe they were more willing to take their chances for a heart attack than they were to risk endometrial cancer. "I think a lot of women are more afraid of endometrial cancer, which they believe they can avoid without treatment, than of osteoporosis, which they feel they probably won't get if they maintain a healthy lifestyle," I said.

"The risk for endometrial cancer is very small," he retorted quickly, "when progestins are given along with estrogen." Then he added, "And most women who get endometrial cancer will have totally curable lesions anyway." As if "a little" endometrial cancer were just a nuisance. . . .

I also remember mentioning to him that I didn't think there

was sufficient evidence for the notion that estrogen treatment prevented heart attacks. In all the many trials, the women who were given and took estrogen treatment were healthier and had fewer known heart disease risks like obesity and sedentary lifestyles than the nonrandomized, nonblinded "control" women who didn't or wouldn't take estrogen. Before he could reply, I continued, "You know that the only double blind randomized controlled studies of conjugated estrogen treatment, studies that were performed in men, showed no prevention of heart attacks and sufficient various complications (pulmonary emboli and thromboses) that the trial was prematurely stopped. Furthermore, there was an unexplained but significantly increased cancer risk, for cancers of all types, in the estrogen-treated men."

"Yes, I know," he said flippantly. "That's why I'm not on estrogen."

It was no use. He was unshakable. His message was truth: *Menopause is an estrogen deficiency disease and must be treated with estrogen.* I have both a clear idea of what I am experiencing as a perimenopausal woman and a scientific understanding of reproductive endocrinology. Yet my experiences are dismissed since they don't fit the current notion. He is not the only one who is certain of the menopause truth. So are other influential physicians: "We suggest estrogen treatment for all women with any stigmata of hormone deprivation."

Yet what do we *really* know? . . . Can we predict a given woman's hormonal changes or experience based on her reproductive life, family history, weight, and exercise? No, we cannot. Instead we ascribe everything that happens in the years before the last period to "estrogen deficiency" and assume that women who don't fit the pattern are imagining things. In reality, we know more about the natural history of AIDS then we do about the menstrual transition!

As I put the phone down, I mused. At least this time I had had a fighting chance to get across a different view of menopause. I knew the booklet editor and he knew of my work. I was even asked to write the chapter. Yet, despite all of these factors in my favor, I was not heard. Although I am chronologically his senior and academically his peer, I had been given no say.

If my voice can be so easily and effectively silenced, are other women likely to be heard?

There you have it: a highly regarded female reproductive scientist, who by virtue of her personal experience, her own scientific studies, and professional knowledge of the relevant literature is dismissed from her task of writing a chapter on a subject she knows very well, the reason being that her conclusions do not fit the prevailing estrogen dogma. The same would be true of other experts whose conclusions differ from the "acceptable" line.

The time has come to clear the air and face reality. That is in part the purpose of this book. Mainstream medicine is firmly entrenched in its belief that menopause connotes the onset of an estrogen deficiency disease that requires estrogen treatment. This, as you will discover, is not only scientifically inaccurate but is a parochial, patriarchal, and narrow-minded view that acts to retard a deeper and more constructive understanding of the problem. In the chapters to come, you will discover a better answer.

Chapter 4

WHAT IS ESTROGEN?

Estrogen and progesterone are closely interrelated in many ways. In a normally functioning premenopausal woman, estrogens are made from progesterone and/or from androgens within the cells of the ovaries. After menopause, estrogens are converted from adrenal-produced androgens, primarily in body fat. Estrogens and progesterone are, in many instances, antagonistic; yet each sensitizes receptors for the other. A key to hormone balance is the knowledge that when estrogen becomes the dominant hormone and progesterone is deficient, the estrogen becomes toxic to the body; thus progesterone has a balancing or mitigating effect on estrogen. There are very, very few Western women truly deficient in estrogen; most become deficient in progesterone. But before we go any further into the estrogen story, there is a semantic problem to clear up. When estrogen was first discovered, researchers assumed it was *the* estrus-producing hormone. As time went on, more types of estrogen were discovered and each one was given a specific chemical name. Thus the word *estrogen* became the name of the *class* of hormones with estrus activity (i.e., proliferation of endometrial cells in preparation for pregnancy). Estrogen is not the name of one hormone, but the name of a group of similar hormones. Let's use apples as an analogy. There is no one apple named apple. There are apples named Winesap, Delicious, and Jonathan, each describing a specific type of apple. In the same sense, there is no estrogen named estrogen. There are estrogens named estrone, estradiol, and estriol. It is common in medical and popular literature about hormones for the author to erroneously refer to estrogen as a hormone that performs this or that function. This is an error that leads to many misconceptions about the estrogens, given the fact that each type of estrogen has a different function in the body. Just as it is possible to make some generalizations about apples, we can make some generalizations about estrogens, but we should avoid thinking they're all the same.

In the case of progesterone, however, we are talking about only one specific hormone. Thus progesterone is both the name of the class and the single member of the class.

Although the word *estrogen* generally refers to the class of hormones produced by the body with similar estrus-like actions, there are also estrogens found outside the body.

*Phyto*estrogens refer to plant compounds with estrogen-like activity. They are usually considerably weaker than one's own estrogens and compete for the same estrogen receptors throughout the body. Thus they have often been used successfully to decrease symptoms of estrogen excess.

*Xeno*estrogens refer to other environmental compounds (usually petrochemical) that generally have very potent estrogen-like activity and thus can be considered very toxic. Though briefly described below, they will be discussed more thoroughly in later chapters.

The fourth type of estrogens we will be discussing are the synthetic estrogens made by the pharmaceutical companies. These have had their molecular structure altered so they can be patented.

Like the xenoestrogens, they tend to be more potent than the body's own estrogens, and more toxic.

An example of synthetic estrogen is diethylstilbestrol (DES). This drug resembles a phytoestrogen called P-anol, found in fennel and anise plants. The DES variation resembles two molecules of P-anol linked end to end and is fully as potent as the body's own estradiol. DES can be inexpensively synthesized and is highly active when taken orally. In the past it was used for regulation of the menstrual cycle, in oral contraceptives, and to prevent premature labor. However, while the P-anol found in plants is harmless when the body is exposed to small quantities, DES has been implicated in certain types of cancer (vaginal and cervical cancer in daughters and testicular cancer in sons of mothers who were given DES during pregnancy). It has been superseded by other, presumably less dangerous compounds. Because estrogen causes fat buildup, DES was also used extensively in beef cattle to fatten them up more quickly for slaughter.

A common feature of estrogenic substances is what is known in chemistry circles as the *phenolated A-ring* of the molecule. (See the appendix on page 356.) We can think of this A-ring as a molecular key that opens the door to some cells. This A-ring, as it is found in estrogens, is not present in progesterone, testosterone, or corticosterone molecules. Most likely, it is this A-ring that distinguishes the estrogenic substances and gives them their specific actions in the body. This same A-ring is common among the xenoestrogens found in petrochemical derivatives (plastics, herbicides, pesticides, industrial by-products such as dioxins) that are pervasively polluting our environment. Some of these are extremely potent estrogenic substances even at nanogram doses. (A nanogram is a billionth of a gram—an inconceivably small amount to most of us.) There is mounting evidence that exposure to xenoestrogens may be a significant causal factor in breast cancer, the decline in male sperm production, testicular cancer, and prostate cancer.

HOW AND WHERE ESTROGENS ARE MADE AND USED IN THE BODY

Estrone, estradiol, and estriol are the three most important estrogens made in the body. Because of their respective position in the biosynthetic pathway, estrone is referred to as E_1, estradiol as E_2, and estriol as E_3. In the nonpregnancy state, estrone and estradiol are produced by the ovary in quantities of only 100 to 200 micrograms per day, and estriol is only a scant by-product of estrone metabolism. During pregnancy, however, the placenta is the major source of estrogens; estriol is produced in milligram quantities, while estrone and estradiol are produced in microgram amounts, with estradiol excreted in the smallest amount. After menopause, estrone continues to be made by conversion of the adrenal steroid, androstenediol, primarily in body fat and muscle cells. The more fat, the more estrone is made. Indeed, some obese women produce more estrogen after menopause than thin premenopausal women. Yet obese women are not immune to the problem of hot flashes.

Estriol made by the placenta is made from a hormone called DHEA (dehydroepiandrosterone), supplied from either the mother or the adrenal cortex of the fetus. Because of fetal participation in estriol formation, estriol measurements can be a sensitive indicator of placenta and/or fetal well-being.

The placenta also becomes the major source of progesterone, producing 300 to 400 milligrams per day during the third trimester. Estriol and progesterone therefore are the major sex steroids present during pregnancy.

ESTROGEN AND CELL DIVISION

Estrogens in general tend to promote cell division, particularly in hormone-sensitive tissue such as the breast and uterine lining. Among the three estrogens, estradiol is most stimulating to the breast and estriol the least. Estradiol is 1,000 times more potent in its effects on breast tissue than estriol. Studies of two decades ago clearly found that overexposure to estradiol (and estrone to a lesser extent) increases one's risk of breast cancer, whereas estriol is protective.

Synthetic ethinyl estradiol, commonly used in estrogen supplements and contraceptives, is even more of a breast cancer risk because it is efficiently absorbed by mouth and slow to be metabolized and excreted. The longer a synthetic estrogen stays in the body, the more opportunity it has to do damage. Since this factor of slow metabolism and excretion is true of all synthetic estrogens, one would think that, in all cases of estrogen supplementation, the natural hormones would be superior.

The brand names of some of the ethinyl estrogens/progestins used as birth control pills are:

Brevicon
Demulen
Desogen
Levlen
Loestrin
Lo/Ovral
Modicon
Neolova
Nordette
Norinyl
Ortho Cyclen
Ortho-Cept

Ortho-Novum
Ovcon
Ovral
Tri-Levlen
Tri-Norinyl
Triphasil

Estriol is the estrogen most beneficial to the vagina, cervix, and vulva. In cases of postmenopausal vaginal dryness and atrophy, which predisposes a woman to vaginitis and cystitis, estriol supplementation would theoretically be the most effective (and safest) estrogen to use.

HOW ESTROGEN AFFECTS A WOMAN'S BODY

Estrogen is responsible for the changes that take place at puberty in girls, such as growth and development of the vagina, uterus, and fallopian tubes. It causes enlargement of the breasts through growth of ducts, stromal tissue, and fat. Estrogen contributes to molding (fatty content) of female body contours and maturation of the skeleton. It is responsible for the growth of underarm and pubic hair and pigmentation of the nipples and areolae.

There are no doubt good evolutionary reasons for some of estrogen's seemingly negative actions on the body such as water retention and weight gain. If we think of estrogen in terms of procreation and survival of the fetus, it would seem advantageous to the baby for the expectant mother to be able, in times of famine, to store body fat. Thus the effects of estrogen include far more than its action in creating the female body form and its stimulation of the uterus and breasts. During times of severe famine when a woman would be nutritionally unable to carry a pregnancy to term, estrogen production decreases to prevent fertility. During times of consistent dietary abundance, however, estrogen's effects are potentially harmful. When women consume considerably more calories than needed, estrogen production increases proportionately to supernormal levels and may set the stage for estrogen dominance syndrome (see below) and exaggerated estrogen decline at menopause. In the United States and most industrially advanced countries, diets are rich in animal fats, sugar, refined starches, and processed foods, providing calories in excess of need and leading to estrogen levels in women twice as high as those in women of the more agrarian third-world countries.

In this context, it is worthwhile to compare the physiological effects of estrogen and progesterone:

Estrogen effects	Progesterone effects
creates proliferative endometrium	maintains secretory endometrium
causes breast stimulation	protects against fibrocystic breasts
increases body fat	helps use fat for energy
salt and fluid retention	natural diuretic
depression and headaches	natural antidepressant
interferes with thyroid hormone	facilitates thyroid hormone action
increases blood clotting	normalizes blood clotting
decreases sex drive	restores sex drive
impairs blood sugar control	normalizes blood sugar levels
loss of zinc and retention of copper	normalizes zinc and copper levels
reduces oxygen levels in all cells	restores proper cell oxygen levels
increases risk of endometrial cancer	prevents endometrial cancer

increases risk of breast cancer	helps prevent breast cancer
slightly restrains osteoclast function	stimulates osteoblast bone building
reduces vascular tone	restores normal vascular tone
increases risk of gallbladder disease	necessary for survival of embryo
increases risk of autoimmune disorders	precursor of corticosteroids

THE ESTROGEN DOMINANCE SYNDROME

It is clear that excess estrogen, when unopposed or unbalanced by progesterone, is not something wholly to be desired. Stated differently, it is clear that many of estrogen's undesirable side effects are effectively prevented by progesterone. I would propose that a new syndrome be recognized: that of *estrogen dominance*. This syndrome, with symptoms familiar to most women in industrialized countries, commonly occurs in the following situations:

1. Estrogen replacement therapy
2. Premenopause (early follicle depletion resulting in a lack of ovulation and thus lack of progesterone well before the onset of menopause)
3. Exposure to xenoestrogens (cause of early follicle depletion)
4. Birth control pills (with excessive estrogen component)
5. Hysterectomy (can induce subsequent ovary dysfunction or atrophy)
6. Postmenopause (especially in overweight women)

Thanks to the nearly universal misconception in Western medicine that estrogen deficiency brings about all menopausal symptoms, it is the custom to prescribe unopposed estrogen for women who do not have a uterus (i.e., have had a hysterectomy). Equally unfortunate is the fact that premenopausal estrogen dominance is simply ignored.

A peculiarity of Western industrialized societies is the prevalence of uterine fibroids, breast and/or uterine cancer, fibrocystic breasts, PMS, ovarian cancer, premenopausal bone loss, and a high incidence of osteoporosis in menopausal women. I believe that most of these are the symptoms of estrogen dominance.

The following is a list of symptoms that can be caused or made worse by estrogen dominance:

Acceleration of the aging process
Allergies
Breast tenderness
Decreased sex drive
Depression
Fatigue
Fibrocystic breasts
Foggy thinking
Headaches
Hypoglycemia
Increased blood clotting (increasing risk of strokes)
Infertility
Irritability
Memory loss
Miscarriage
Osteoporosis
Premenopausal bone loss
PMS
Thyroid dysfunction mimicking hypothyroidism
Uterine cancer
Uterine fibroids
Water retention, bloating

Fat gain, especially around the abdomen, hips, and thighs
Gallbladder disease
Autoimmune disorders such as lupus erythematosus and thyroiditis
  and possibly Sjögren's disease

THE MYTH OF ESTROGEN IN HORMONE REPLACEMENT THERAPY

Most physicians are attempting to push hormone replacement therapy (HRT) featuring synthetic estrogens and progestins onto *all* menopausal women. Their enthusiasm for these drugs, however, is not backed up by the facts. Let's examine some of the claims being made for HRT.

The chief argument for postmenopausal estrogen supplementation is the deeply ingrained assumption of estrogen deficiency after menopause. This is touted in all pharmaceutical estrogen ads, many medical texts, lay publications, and by mainstream medical practitioners. Women are reminded that their mood swings, depressions, hot flashes, vaginal dryness, loss of sex drive, and accelerating osteoporosis are indisputable evidence of estrogen deficiency. Menopause is treated as the onset of an estrogen deficiency disease. Indeed, Dr. Elaine Jolly, Director of the Reproductive Endocrinology Clinic at the Ottawa General Hospital and editor of the Menopause Consensus Committee of the Society of Obstetricians and Gynecologists of Canada (SOGC) believes that "menopause is an endocrine deficient state that should be managed with estrogen." But is this true?

It is true that menopause is known to be associated with decreasing estrogen levels, but what is not known is whether these decreased levels of estrogen do in fact cause all the symptoms of menopause. Carolyn DeMarco, M.D. (who has been in practice over twenty years specializing in women's health issues, is the author of the book *Take Charge of Your Body* and a widely respected contributor to other publications and health councils) states that "there is no direct proof that estrogen lack causes heart disease or other ailments associated with the menopause." Germaine Greer, well-known feminist and author of *The Change,* writes that "the proponents of HRT have never proved that there is an estrogen deficiency, nor have they explained the mechanism by which the therapy of choice effected its miracles. They have taken the improper course of defining a disease from its therapy."

Dr. Jerilynn Prior, researcher and professor of endocrinology at the University of British Columbia in Vancouver, B.C., Canada, points out that no study proving the relationship between estrogen deficiency and menopausal symptoms and related diseases has yet been done. "Instead," says Dr. Prior, "a notion has been put forward that since estrogen levels go down, this is the most important change and explains all the things that may or may not be related to menopause. So estrogen treatment at this stage of our understanding is premature. This is a kind of backwards science. It leads to ridiculous ideas—like calling a headache an aspirin deficiency disease."

Western women tend to have a 10- to 15-year period prior to menopause when they are estrogen dominant and suffering from estrogen dominance symptoms, and some doctors are giving them more estrogen. Something is terribly wrong here!

While it is common experience that estrogen supplementation relieves many women of certain postmenopausal symptoms, it is not at all clearly established that estrogen deficiency per se was the cause. For example, none of the estrogen proponents have bothered to check progesterone levels before and after menopause. As Dr. Prior has pointed out, during menopause, progesterone decreases to $1/120$ of baseline levels whereas estrogen decreases only to one-half to one-third of premenopausal baseline levels. Would it not be wise to consider the progesterone loss effect when evaluating postmenopausal symptoms and related conditions such as osteoporosis, heart disease, depression, and loss of sex drive?

Dr. Graham Colditz, associate professor at the Harvard Medical School, is an eminent and respected authority on the breast cancer risks of estrogens. In a talk he gave in San Francisco at the February 1994 meeting of the American Association for the Advancement of Science, he included an interesting graph of pre- and postmenopausal plasma levels of estrone plus estradiol. His graph showed typical *pre*menopausal levels to be 2.35 and untreated *post*menopausal levels to be 2 (the scale dimensions were not identified). This is a drop of only 15 percent—just enough to

ESTROGEN AND PROGESTERONE RATIOS

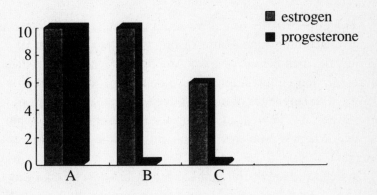

Figure 3: A = balance of estrogen and progesterone during the secretory phase of a normal menstrual cycle

B = relative production of estrogen and progesterone during an anovulatory premenopausal menstrual cycle

C = relative production of estrogen and progesterone after menopause

allow menstruation to stop. But 85 percent of a woman's estrogen is still present!

The graph on page 45 depicts the relative balance of estrogen and progesterone during a normal menstrual cycle, an anovulatory cycle, and after menopause.

In this graph, estrogen and progesterone are assumed to be in balance during the secretory phase of a normal menstrual cycle. In an anovulatory menstrual cycle, estrogen remains the same and progesterone production drops to very low levels. After menopause, estrogen production decreases 40 to 60 percent and progesterone remains at very low levels. Thus in anovulatory *and* menopausal conditions, estrogen dominance persists.

WHAT ARE "NORMAL" ESTROGEN LEVELS?

Another peculiarity of the Western mainstream medical practitioner concerning menopause disorders is the ignorance of the worldwide menopause picture. Among the less industrialized, more agrarian cultures, menopause complaints are minor or unknown. The languages of many of these cultures have no word for hot flashes. The advent of menopause in these cultures is not a portent of health problems. Why is this so little known in North America?

Dr. Peter Ellison of Harvard University has developed a way to measure women's ovarian hormones using saliva, making it relatively simple to study hormone levels in their natural settings. He has reported his findings of ovarian hormone levels in various populations of distinct genetic, ecological, and cultural backgrounds. He found that in Western populations premenopausal estrogen levels represent a high extreme of the spectrum and should be considered abnormal. Further, he suggests that these abnormal levels may relate to the current epidemic of breast and ovarian cancer.

Dr. Ellison believes there is a direct link between hormone levels and energy balance, meaning the balance between dietary energy intake and energy expended in work. A negative energy balance (a woman who does a lot of physical work and doesn't have enough to eat) will tend to lower hormone levels, presumably protecting her against the higher energy requirements of pregnancy. A positive energy balance (a woman who doesn't get much physical exercise and eats more than she needs) raises hormone levels. Ellison conjectures that the high hormone levels found in Western cultures are a reflection of overeating and underexercising common in these populations. Further, Ellison suggests the higher ovarian function common in Western populations results in a proportionately greater fall in hormone levels at menopause, and this may account for the greater incidence and severity of menopausal symptoms seen. In nonindustrialized populations, the discrepancy between pre- and postmenopausal hormone levels is considerably less than in industrialized populations. Remember, postmenopausal estrogen levels do not drop to zero, they merely drop to the level that will not produce a blood-rich uterine lining to be shed. If Dr. Ellison's hypothesis is correct, it may mean that prevention of menopausal symptoms could be accomplished by eating less and getting more exercise. It would be very useful to conduct a study of Western menopausal women to find out if there is a correlation between menopausal symptoms and various groups of women who differ substantially in terms of exercise and diet.

Our dietary problem includes not only the fact of excess calories but also the nutritional quality of our foods. A diet rich in fatty meats, sugar, refined carbohydrates, and processed foods is quite different from a plant-based diet high in fiber, nutrients, phytoestrogens, antioxidants, and complex carbohydrates. Such diets directly affect hormone production. In an article titled "Oestrogen Overdose" by Gail Vines in the September 1994 issue of *British Vogue,* Lyliane Rosetta, physiologist at the Université René Descartes in Paris, found that estrogen and progesterone levels fell in women who switched to a low-fat, high-fiber, plant-based diet with more legumes even though they did not gain or lose weight and ate as many calories as women in the control group who had a traditional Western diet, high in fat and simple carbohydrates.

It is also interesting to note that as one researches the more authoritative texts on hormones, one finds a vastly different view of the supposed estrogen "deficiency" status of postmenopausal women from that promoted by the pharmaceutical companies. The following quote from *Novak's Textbook of Gynecology* (11th edition, Williams & Wilkins, 1987) is representative of the views of the experts who are not being paid to promote estrogen:

> Thus it would seem that although menopausal women do have an estrogen milieu that is lower than that necessary for reproduction, it is not negligible or absent but is perhaps satisfactory for maintenance of support tissues. The menopause could then be regarded as a physiologic phenomenon that is protective in nature, protective from the undesirable reproduction and the associated growth stimuli.

In plain language, this means that, in most menopausal women, estrogen levels are below that necessary for pregnancy but sufficient for other normal body functions, as well as being a whole lot safer. The estrogen "deficiency" hypothesis as an explanation of postmenopausal symptoms or health problems is thus not supported by the facts of estrogen blood levels, by worldwide ecologic surveys, or by endocrinology experts.

Menopause per se should be regarded as a normal physiologic

adjustment reflecting a benign change in a woman's biological life away from childbearing and onward to a period of new personal power and fulfillment. The Western perception of menopause as a threshold of undesirable symptoms and progressive illness due to estrogen deficiency is an error unsupported by fact. More accurately, we should view our menopause problem as an abnormality brought about by industrialized cultures' deviation from a healthy lifestyle.

Chapter 5

HORMONE BALANCE, XENOBIOTICS, AND FUTURE GENERATIONS

Throughout this book I will be referring repeatedly to xenobiotics or xenoestrogens, foreign substances originating outside the body that have hormone-like and estrogen-like activity in the body, and thus a profound impact on hormone balance. I will use the term "xenobiotics" as a generic reference to substances with a hormone-like effect on the body and "xenoestrogens" to specifically describe those with an estrogenic effect on the body.

Nearly all xenobiotics are petrochemically based, meaning "derived from petroleum oil." We live in a pervasively petrochemical world. Our machines run on petroleum fuels, many of our buildings are heated with petroleum oil, and thousands, maybe millions of products, including plastics, microchips, medicines, clothing, foods, soaps, pesticides, and even perfumes, are made from petrochemicals or contain them. While these substances have undeniably improved our quality of life, the price we pay is pervasive petrochemical pollution of the air, water, soil, and our bodies.

The legacy of this pollution in living creatures, including humans, includes an epidemic of reproductive abnormalities, including steadily increasing numbers of cancers of the reproductive tract, infertility, low sperm counts, and the feminization of males. Estrogen is the female hormone and we are awash in a petrochemical sea of xenoestrogens. The potential consequences of this overexposure are staggering, especially considering that one of the consequences is passing on reproductive abnormalities to offspring.

And don't think I am being unduly alarmist here. Theo Colborn, Ph.D., senior scientist and manager of the Wildlife & Contaminants Project at the World Wildlife Fund, closely follows the research of others and coordinates the big picture. She arranged a gathering of 21 wildlife experts to discuss the topic of "Environmentally Induced Alterations in Development: A Focus on Wildlife." This meeting inspired an understanding in all who attended of the enormity and importance of their various individual observations of increasing reproductive abnormalities in adults and embryos in a large number of wildlife species, decreasing populations, and the implications for humans. It led to a remarkable consensus statement alerting the world to the dangers of environmental petrochemicals that "mimic and/or interfere with female and male hormones, thereby modifying development and reproduction." Such chemicals are now referred to as "xenobiotics." The majority of xenobiotics mimic the action of estrogen, thus the common use of the term "xenoestrogen."

By-products of manufacturing processes that use chlorine and compounds formed when chlorine interacts with organic matter, called organochlorines, are such a serious threat to our health and the environment, both as potent carcinogens (dioxins and PCBs) and as xenobiotics, that President William Clinton, the World Health Organization (WHO), and the United States-Canadian Joint Commission (IJC) have called for a phaseout of the use of chlorine and chlorinated compounds.

There is truly no way we can live in a Western culture at this time and altogether avoid coming into contact with petrochemical pollutants. However, we can minimize our exposure to those that behave like estrogens, and I'll tell you how as I discuss the sources of xenobiotics. But first, let's examine some of the biochemistry behind xenobiotics, as well as the evidence that they are profoundly affecting the sexual and reproductive health of future generations.

TURNING ON THE HORMONE SWITCH

Why do some petrochemicals behave as potent estrogens? Something in their molecular structure contains the basic "key" that fits in the hormone receptor "ignition" of the cell, switching on hormonal action. John McLachlan, Ph.D., who was chief of the National Institute of Environmental Health Sciences (NIEHS) and is now director of the Tulane/Xavier Center for Bioenvironmental Research, explains that it is difficult to track these chemicals by traditional toxicology methods. Their effect may not show up until the next generation, and furthermore, we cannot judge a petrochemical's hormonal potential by any specific attribute of their molecular structure. McLachlan has therefore suggested the development of a "functional toxicology," in which chemicals are defined more by their function than by their chemistry. He recommends an array of panels made up of cells containing receptors for the hormones in question. Chemicals could be tested for their ability to occupy, activate, or turn off cell receptors.

McLachlan's vision of the future is that this information be included along with chemical information such as melting point, molecular weight, and solubility. Personally I'd like to see these effects listed on every can of bug spray, every box and bottle of weed killer, on the sides of the trucks that spray chemicals on lawns, on every box of detergent or tub and tile cleaner that contains nonylphenols, and everywhere else in our environment that we're exposed to these chemicals. If food manufacturers have to list calories, grams of fat, and sodium on their labels, shouldn't chemical manufacturers be obliged to let us know when their product may cause reproductive abnormalities in our offspring?

As you remember, synthetic drugs tend to be far more potent than their natural derivatives. The xenoestrogens have the same property. In their estrogenic activity, these estrogens are considerably more potent than the estrogen made by the ovaries. In their effect on fish, some of them have been found to be potent estrogenic substances even at nanogram doses. A nanogram is a billionth of a gram, which is roughly the same proportion as a grain of sand to an Olympic swimming pool. If we extrapolate this to the human body, the amount of a xenoestrogen necessary to have an estrogenic effect is inconceivably small. A popular argument by those who feel that xenoestrogens are harmless is that the amounts we're exposed to from any one source are generally very tiny. What these people fail to take into account is the multitude of ways in which we are exposed to these substances every day.

McLachlan explains the various effects of hormonal mimics with the following diagram:

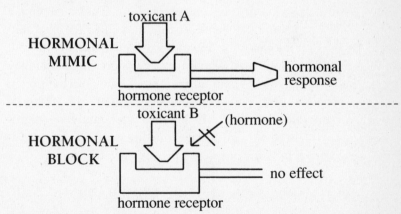

Figure 4: Some hormonal mimics (e.g., progestins and xenoestrogens) activate the receptor to stimulate the hormone effect while others will occupy the receptor and block the natural hormone from doing its work.

THE CANARY IN THE COAL MINE?

Xenobiotics come from many sources and have a multitude of biochemical effects on living creatures. Thanks to testing done by a wide array of scientists, we know beyond a doubt that xenobiotics are threatening the survival of many birds, reptiles, and mammals in North America. We would be wise to pay attention to what's happening with these animals. Miners used to take a canary in a cage down into the mine with them. If the sensitive canary suddenly keeled over and died, they hightailed it out of the mine, knowing the air was poisonous and that soon they would be keeling over. The many animal species more sensitive than humans that are effectively being exterminated by overdoses of xenobiotics could be a large environmental version of the canary in the cage.

When the superb *Science News* writer Janet Raloff broke the xenobiotic story to the general public back in the summer of 1993, in an article called "EcoCancers," she pointed out that scientists have known about the effects of xenobiotics since the early 1970s. She followed that first article with two others in January of 1994. Her well-researched, articulate, and compelling articles inspired a spate of newspaper and magazine articles, as well as TV and radio shows about xenobiotics, which in turn inspired testimony in front of Congress from a scientist who informed congressmen that they were "half the men their grandfathers were," thanks to the prevalence of xenoestrogens in the environment. Now it's a question of whether corporate America, which relies so heavily on petrochemicals, will heed this information in favor of future generations or ignore it in favor of today's profits.

THE IMPACT ON FUTURE GENERATIONS

There is much evidence that xenobiotics harm future generations. Studies done at the University of California, Davis, show that seagulls whose eggs are injected with estradiol hatch chicks that show the same birth defects as those exposed to DDT: chemically castrated males with feminized gonads and females with overdeveloped ovaries. Michael Fry, Ph.D., a professor at the University of California, Davis, Department of Avian Sciences, researches the toxic effects of airborne and waterborne organochlorine pesticides on the development and reproduction of birds. Some of the abnormalities he has found in birds exposed to xenobiotics include clubbed feet, crossed bills, huge thyroid glands, nests with more than the normal number of eggs (laid by more than one bird), a surplus of females, female-female pairing, feminization of male reproductive tracts, ovarian cortical tissue in testes, abnormal persistence of oviducts in males, and general failure to thrive. Experimental injection of organochlorines into gull eggs reproduced these abnormalities. Eggshell thinning in gulls occurs in eggs laid by adult birds that have been exposed to estrogenic chemicals while still embryos.

Scientists at the University of Florida in Gainesville found that both male and female alligators born after a pesticide spill exposed their parents to a pesticide similar to DDT called dicofol have abnormally high levels of estrogen and low levels of testosterone. Additionally, the females have abnormal ovaries and follicles described as "burned out," and the males have abnormally small penises. Since the pesticide spill in Florida's Lake Apopka in 1980, the number of young alligators has been reduced by 90 percent. The implication is that the alligators there are no longer capable of reproducing.

In a May 1993 article in *Lancet,* researchers in Scotland and Denmark hypothesized that xenobiotics are responsible for a steadily declining sperm count in men. According to Niels Skakkebaek of the University of Copenhagen, sperm counts have dropped by more than 50 percent since 1940. Meanwhile, the rate of testicular cancer in the United States and Europe has more than tripled in the past 50 years and reproductive abnormalities such as undescended testicles have become increasingly common. The decline of sperm counts began at the same time that "better living through chemistry" became the national anthem of big business in America and Europe and we began being carelessly exposed to petrochemical pollutants.

SAFE LIVING IN A SEA OF ESTROGENS

Xenoestrogens, in addition to being highly estrogenic, are fat-soluble and nonbiodegradable. Because of the widespread use of petrochemical products in our society, they are difficult to avoid, but we can significantly reduce our exposure. The major source of oral intake of xenoestrogens is by way of animal fats, particularly red meat and dairy fats. In addition to the fact that these animals are often given estrogenic substances to fatten them up for market, they are also exposed when they eat grains that have been sprayed with pesticides. The xenoestrogens accumulate in their fat. For every 15 pounds of grain a steer eats, you get one pound of beef, so there's a relatively high amount of these pesticides in the meat of these animals. Anyone who eats meat and dairy products is eating these compounds and they are all potent estrogens. They accumulate in our fatty tissues (breast, brain, and liver) and cause estrogen dominance, with all of its attendant symptoms.

Reproductive organ changes caused by xenobiotics have been reported by a long list of scientists in North America and Europe in everything from wrens and panthers to sturgeons and turtles. DDT, PCBs, or dioxins are often found in the tissues of these animals. But these are just three of the most potent xenobiotics that stay in the body for a lifetime. Other xenobiotics may not stay in the body but will have their effect passing through the body. The majority of other xenobiotics come to us through petrochemical pollution, including some from rather bizarre sources.

Sumpter and Charles Tyler of Brunel University in Uxbridge, England, exposed trout to effluent (treated sewage) at a variety of sites. After exposure, the fish tested positive for high amounts of a chemical called vitellogenin, indicating they had been exposed to an excess of estrogen. When the Tylers were unable to find an industrial source for these xenoestrogens, they finally theorized that it must be coming from the urine of women taking birth control pills containing the synthetic estrogen ethinylestradiol (EE). When they tested this hypothesis in the laboratory by exposing the fish to EE, they found that nanogram amounts of this estrogen could cause vitellogenin levels to spike in the trout. The implications of this discovery are immense, because synthetic estrogens are being dumped into waterways all over Europe and North America and have entered the food chain.

In the process of uncovering the source of the estrogen effect in these fish, the Tylers also discovered another ubiquitous source of xenoestrogens: nonylphenols, breakdown products of surfactants commonly used in detergents (including dishwashing liquids), cosmetics and other toiletries, and pesticides and herbicides. Although nonylphenols are not as potent as EEs, they are dumped in our waterways in much higher quantities. This is a good reason to buy "green" (i.e., environmentally safe) products when you go to the supermarket. Ironically, nonylphenols are found in the spermicides used for birth control in diaphragm jellies, on condoms, and in vaginal gels to facilitate dispersal. This directly exposes the vagina and cervix to xenoestrogens.

Even without the nonylphenols added to them, nearly all petrochemical pesticides, herbicides, and fungicides are potent xenobiotics. Billions of pounds of these substances are applied to our fruits and vegetables every year, and many of them don't go away; when you eat the fruit or vegetable you generally get a dose, albeit a small one, of pesticides along with it. This is why I suggest everyone eat organic fruits and vegetables as much as possible. The more we, as consumers, demand organic produce, the more likely it is to be grown that way. When farmers first switched back to organic methods a few decades ago, the produce tended to be small and not very nice looking compared to what we were used to. Now that organic farmers have had a couple of decades to practice, organic produce tends to be just as beautiful, even more tasty, and, because it is grown in rich, healthy soil, more nutritious than its contaminated counterpart.

We also use petrochemical pesticides in our homes in the form of bug spray, as well as on our lawns and gardens. There is absolutely no need to use these poisons around your home. There are a wealth of excellent books out on simple, easy, and cost-effective methods of organic gardening and pest control. (See "Recommended Reading" on page 331.) Many communities in the United States have city- or county-sponsored classes on organic gardening and pest control.

Another nearly universal source of xenoestrogens is plastics. Some types of plastic shed xenoestrogens when they are heated. Since it would be nearly impossible to figure out which plastics shed xenoestrogens, the best approach is to assume they all do and behave accordingly. Don't routinely drink hot beverages from plastic cups and don't routinely microwave your food in plastic containers. If you don't buy coffee in plastic cups and frozen food in plastic containers, the manufacturers will eventually catch on and stop making them that way.

XENOESTROGENS AND FUTURE GENERATIONS

Excess estrogen exposure in humans in the first trimester of pregnancy can affect fetal sexual development. We first learned this painful lesson via the sons and daughters of women given DES (diethylstilbestrol) during pregnancy. DES is a synthetic estrogen that was given to women to prevent miscarriage, to treat breast cancer, and to reduce the symptoms of menopause. Between 1948 and 1971 it was taken by two to six million women in the United States and Europe. Some 50,000 pounds of DES were also dumped into livestock feed to fatten them up for market until it was banned in 1979 because it was showing up in supermarket beef in measurable amounts. (There are rumors that DES is still used illegally in livestock feed.) In the early 1970s, researchers looking for links to a high incidence of cervical cancers in young women traced it to their mothers, who were prescribed DES during pregnancy to prevent miscarriage. Further research has shown that the use of DES in pregnancy is also linked to testicular cancer in males, as well as infertility, birth defects, and other reproductive problems in both sexes.

Lurking as an unknown factor in the later development of one's sexual preference is the possibility of fetal influence by the xenobiotics found in our petrochemically polluted environment. Having now mentioned this factor in a number of talks I've given, I realize it may not be a politically correct position, but nevertheless I feel it is an important factor to consider. If xenobiotics can blur the distinctions between the sexes in seagulls and alligators at nanogram levels, how farfetched is it to speculate that the same pollutants may be affecting humans in a similar fashion? Recently it has been found that daughters of mothers who had been given DES during pregnancy are not only more likely to develop vaginal and cervical cancer, but also to become bisexual or lesbians as adults.

I believe xenoestrogens are affecting our children in profound ways. Girls used to begin menstruation around age 16. Now they may start menstruating as early as 10 years old. We have come to think of this as normal. It's not. Some scientists claim this is a sign of better nutrition. My suspicion is that this early onset of puberty is caused by exposure to the xenoestrogens so prevelant in every part of our environment, from our meat supply to the air we breathe, combined with diets sadly lacking in the whole foods that contain the protective phytoestrogens. The long-term consequences of early menstruation are a longer lifetime exposure to estrogen, with an increased risk of hormone-driven cancers such as breast and uterine cancer.

It's time for us to wake up and pay heed to these warnings for the sake of future generations. You can play your part in protecting our grandchildren and great-grandchildren in the same ways you can protect yourself: by refusing to use pesticides, minimizing your use of plastics, purchasing hormone-free meat and organic produce, using "green" products for detergents and household cleaners, and, in general, using "natural" products in favor of petrochemical products. I realize using these types of products costs slightly more, but it seems a small price to pay to insure our future reproductive health.

Chapter 6

WHAT IS NATURAL PROGESTERONE?

Progesterone is a primary hormone of fertility and pregnancy. Fertility has always fascinated humankind. Fertility and pregnancy symbols, rites, and icons abound in all cultures throughout human history. It is only since Old Testament times that fertility and pregnancy have *not* been a source of religion and worship in the Western world. Woman's ability to bleed every month without dying, as well as her ability to bring new life into the world, was regarded as sacred. These miraculous abilities no doubt inspired the goddess worship prevalent throughout the world for so much of early human history.

The regular occurrence of natural breeding times, annually in some animals and monthly in human females, provided the first real understanding of male and female roles in reproduction. These cycles of fertility were recognized several millennia before Christ. The early Greeks provided us with the medical word *oestrus* or *estrus,* which to them meant "frenzy," and to us now means a cyclic period of sexual activity. Other cultures used their words for heat to describe the fruitful breeding times of most mammals and human females. The causes of these cyclic occurrences of fertility and bleeding were unknown to the Greeks and still regarded as sacred.

With the ascendancy of patriarchal cultures, females were assigned a different role in reproduction. Through the Middle Ages in Europe women were considered the receptacle for the germinating seed of man. One has to wonder about the origin of this belief, since the female contribution to offspring is obvious in humans by simply observing the many children who strongly resemble their mothers. Not until the mid-1800s did scientists acknowledge that the female provided an equal share of the inherited characteristics of her offspring.

In 1866, Gregor Mendel, an obscure Austrian monk, published his paper on the hybridization of peas describing the equal importance of male and female factors to inherited characteristics of succeeding plant generations. Despite the impetus stemming from the independent but simultaneous publications in 1858 by Charles Darwin and A. R. Wallace, as well as Darwin's superb and very successful book *Origin of Species* (1859), all dealing with inherited factors of selection as the keystone of evolution, the prevailing view of male dominance in Western culture was still so great that Mendel's work was essentially ignored at the time. However, these genetic principles were rediscovered a generation later in 1900 by three scientists, Hugo de Vries, C. G. Correns, and Erich Tschermak-Seysenegg, each working independently in different countries.

THE DISCOVERY AND USE OF PROGESTERONE

Not only did the science of genetics make a quantum leap during the early 1900s, but so also did the science of the biochemistry of reproduction. In 1900, the role of ovaries in hormonal control of the female reproductive system was established. In 1926 the hormone we now call estrogen was discovered in the urine of menstruating women, and scientists next observed that the concentration of the hormone varied with the phase of the menstrual cycle.

Many early researchers had correctly postulated that the ovary produced two hormonal substances. As early as 1897, researchers suggested that the small yellowish bodies (the corpora lutea) found on the ovary surface of pregnant females must serve a necessary function during pregnancy. In 1903 it was shown that destruction of the corpora lutea in pregnant rabbits caused abortion. With the discovery of the importance of the corpus luteum in hormone production, the second hormone was soon identified. In 1929, the existence of the corpus luteum hormone was finally established, was proven to be necessary for a successful pregnancy, and thus was given the name progesterone (i.e., "pro-gestation").

As you'll recall, we now know that at birth ovaries contain hundreds of thousands of tiny sacs called follicles, each holding a potential egg (ovum). Each menstrual cycle results in the activation of 150 or so follicles to bring their egg to a mature state. When one of these follicles has moved to the outer surface of the ovary and released its egg (ovulation), it becomes the corpus luteum, the central manufacturing plant for progesterone.

For several years progesterone research was hampered by the small amount of progesterone that could be obtained from sows' ovaries. However, by the late 1930s, the placenta was found to synthesize progesterone in relatively large amounts, and this led to the harvesting of placentas after childbirth and quick-freezing them for extraction of progesterone in quantities sufficient for experimental work and clinical application. Then, in 1939, Russell E. Marker devised a method to convert sarsasapogenin, a sapogenin found in the sarsaparilla plant, into a progesterone-like compound. Soon thereafter he was able to convert disogenin from the wild yam (*Dioscorea villosa*) into progesterone with an excellent yield

of 40 percent. With this method of production the price of progesterone fell from $80 per gram to $.50 per gram.

Progesterone was found to be a fat-soluble compound that,
when given orally, was relatively ineffective because most of it is
quickly disposed of via the liver. When dissolved in vegetable oil
and given by injection, progesterone is rapidly absorbed and thoroughly effective. Unfortunately, intramuscular injections in
amounts over 100 milligrams proved to be locally irritating and
painful, somewhat limiting its use. Physicians attuned to the intricacies of hormone balance, however, found progesterone to be remarkably effective in treating patients with what is now called
PMS, treating ovarian cysts, and preventing threatened abortion.
Progesterone is also well absorbed when given as a suppository in
the rectum or vagina, and these methods of giving progesterone
are still commonly used in Europe and England, although most
women dislike their messiness. Katherina Dalton, M.D., of London has become world-famous for her highly successful treatments of PMS with transrectal progesterone.

In the early 1950s, active estrogen- and progesterone-like substances called phytoestrogens and phytoprogesterones were found
in thousands of plant varieties. As mentioned above, the sterol
diosgenin is abundant in a variety of tropical wild yams with the
Latin name *Dioscorea,* and can be converted economically into
exactly the same molecule as human progesterone. (The wild yam
is a different species from the yams we eat in North America. Our
yams are not even true yams and have little to no plant steroid activity.) Furthermore, it was soon discovered that the diosgenin-
derived progesterone could then be used inexpensively to create
synthetic variations of progesterone (progestins) with potent
progestational activity, as well as synthetic estrogens and testosterone, all with profitable commercial application. More recently,
diosgenin is being extracted from soybeans, one of the largest
agricultural crops in America.

Man-made hormones not found in nature are far more profitable for the pharmaceutical companies than natural hormones because, unlike natural substances, they can be patented. Thus pharmaceutical funding for progesterone research early on veered in the direction of creating new and patentable synthetic progesterone analogs made from the yam-derived natural progesterone. This led to the introduction of new classes of so-called progestational agents that lasted longer in the body and were more effective when taken orally. Such agents are referred to as progestins, progestogens, and gestagens, all meaning the same thing: "any synthetically derived compound with the ability to sustain the human secretory endometrium." The progestational agents do not provide the full spectrum of natural progesterone's biological activity, nor are they as safe. Despite their long list of safety concerns (see page 86), progestins have become popular because of their effectiveness in birth control and as protection against the estrogen-induced risk of endometrial cancer. It is a sad commentary on the pursuit of profit over women's well-being that the pharmaceutical companies take perfectly good natural hormones that our bodies know and can use and alter them, creating synthetic compounds with similar hormonal effects but toxic side effects. Research on natural progesterone has in the past two decades been essentially nonexistent. Thus does industrial profit influence the path of science.

The pharmaceutical companies that sell these patented prescription products have been remarkably successful in confusing doctors about the meaning of "progesterone." The typical doctor thinks that the synthetic products are actually progesterone! Since the progestins carry the risk of a long list of undesirable and potentially dangerous side effects, doctors have become leery of prescribing what they think is the natural progesterone, which has no known side effects. This error of confusing the specific hormone, progesterone, with the synthetic progestins is rampant throughout the medical literature. Numerous authors and articles list the multiple health risks of the progestins as "progesterone" risks and the unwary reader becomes progressively more misinformed.

Ignorance about progesterone began years ago and was well under way when I graduated from medical school in 1955. For some time in my medical practice as a family physician, I was one of those doctors who prescribed estrogen. I had graduated from the University of Minnesota Medical School, completed a residency at Minneapolis General Hospital, spent a good portion of a year in practice with a wizard physician in a small town in Minnesota, completed two interesting years in the Pacific area as a medical officer in the U. S. Navy, and, in 1959, opened my own general practice of medicine in Mill Valley, California. I felt confident and well trained. I was good at explaining the workings of birth control pills and had become an editor of a monthly medical journal. But I was still troubled by those women who came to me with premenstrual bloating, water retention, and emotional problems who told me that their previous doctor (usually an older, highly intelligent one back East) had treated them successfully with "progesterone shots." My treatments of diuretics, birth control hormones, or mild tranquilizers were usually unsuccessful, and our local pharmacies no longer carried injectable progesterone. The first modern era of natural progesterone had been short-lived and had come and gone before my time, swamped by the flood of synthetic hormones.

Recently, however, the advantages of natural progesterone have again become evident and its use in clinical situations is growing due to an increasing dissatisfaction among women taking the synthetic HRT regimens. Many physicians who once left the intricacies of hormone balance to gynecologists and endocrinologist consultants are (spurred by the demands of their patients) returning to their textbooks to relearn the lessons they have so long ignored. I receive dozens of letters and phone calls *daily* from women, doctors, and other health professionals in North America and Europe who have used natural progesterone with great success in treating a wide variety of female health problems. There is a quiet revolution going on among those who have discovered natural progesterone and are happily and healthily using it.

EXACTLY WHAT IS PROGESTERONE?

Progesterone is one of two main hormones, the other being estrogen, made by the ovaries of menstruating women. As described above, progesterone is made by the corpus luteum of the ovary, starting just before ovulation and increasing rapidly after ovulation. It is the major female reproductive hormone during the latter two weeks of the menstrual cycle. Progesterone is necessary for the survival of the fertilized ovum, the resulting embryo, and the fetus throughout gestation, when production of progesterone is taken over by the placenta.

To review, in the ovaries, progesterone is the precursor of estrogen. Progesterone is also made in smaller amounts by the adrenal glands in both sexes and by the testes in males. It is a precursor of testosterone and of all the important adrenal cortical hormones. Progesterone is made from the sterol pregnenolone, which is in turn made from cholesterol, which is made from acetate, a product of the breakdown of sugar and fat in the body. Within all cells of the body (except the red blood cells) are tiny power units called mitochondria, which convert cholesterol to pregnenolone, which in turn is converted to progesterone in the ovaries and adrenals. Progesterone is carried in the bloodstream where it is either used by the body or, as it passes through the liver, is excreted.

From progesterone are derived not only the other sex hormones, including the estrogens, but also the corticosteroids, which are essential for stress response, sugar and electrolyte balance, and blood pressure, not to mention survival. With progesterone as a precursor to so many other hormones, it's easy to see why a progesterone deficiency can cause such a wide range of problems.

In short, the three major functions of progesterone are:

1. to promote the survival and development of the embryo and fetus
2. to provide a broad range of intrinsic biologic effects
3. to act as a precursor of other steroid hormones

Progesterone is a central factor in the biosynthesis of other hormones, but its many functions in the body are far more extensive. (For a complete biochemical drawing of the many roles of progesterone, see the appendix on page 356.)

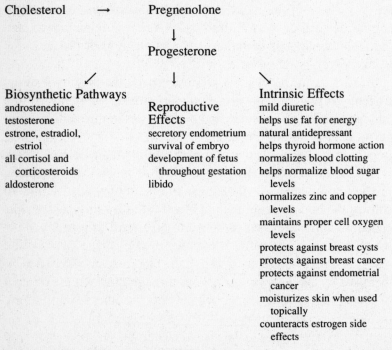

Cholesterol ⟶ Pregnenolone

↓

Progesterone

↓

Biosynthetic Pathways
androstenedione
testosterone
estrone, estradiol,
    estriol
all cortisol and
    corticosteroids
aldosterone

Reproductive Effects
secretory endometrium
survival of embryo
development of fetus
    throughout gestation
libido

Intrinsic Effects
mild diuretic
helps use fat for energy
natural antidepressant
helps thyroid hormone action
normalizes blood clotting
helps normalize blood sugar
    levels
normalizes zinc and copper
    levels
maintains proper cell oxygen
    levels
protects against breast cysts
protects against breast cancer
protects against endometrial
    cancer
moisturizes skin when used
    topically
counteracts estrogen side
    effects

Figure 5: The multiple roles of natural progesterone.

THE CYCLE OF PROGESTERONE PRODUCTION

The levels of progesterone in a woman's body rise and fall dramatically with her monthly cycles. With the development of the corpus luteum and ovulation, the ovarian production of progesterone rapidly rises from two to three milligrams per day to an average of 22 milligrams per day, peak production being as high as 30 milligrams per day a week or so after ovulation. After ten or twelve days, if fertilization does not occur, ovarian production of progesterone falls dramatically. It is this sudden decline in progesterone levels (as well as estrogen levels) that triggers menstruation, i.e. the shedding of the secretory endometrium (the lining of the uterus), leading to a renewal of the entire menstrual cycle.

PROGESTERONE AND PROCREATION

Progesterone is the hormone that makes possible the survival of the fertilized egg. It maintains the lining of the uterus, which the fertilized egg will attach to and from which the germinating egg and the resultant embryo will gain sustenance during its first stages of growth. As might be expected, the surge of progesterone at the time of ovulation is a source of sex drive, the urge to procreate, by which is meant the sexual drive to bring egg and sperm together. (Doesn't it make sense that Mother Nature would connect sex drive to the hormone that comes at ovulation?)

In pregnancy, progesterone is necessary to prevent the premature shedding of the uterine lining. Any drop in progesterone level or blockage of its receptor sites at this time will result in the loss of the embryo (abortion). This in fact is the action of the antiprogesterone compound and abortifacient RU-486.

As the placenta develops, it assumes and progressively increases the production of progesterone for the duration of the gestation period until the birth of the baby. During the third trimester, the placenta is producing progesterone at the rate of 300 to 400 milligrams per day, an astoundingly high level for hormone production, which is usually measured in *micrograms* per day. It is interesting to note that many women say that aside from the physical discomfort of carrying all that extra weight and the constriction of organs such as the bladder, they never felt better than in their third trimester of pregnancy, when progesterone production is very high!

At birth the level of progesterone production drops suddenly, causing postpartum depression in some women. Postpartum depression, should it occur, can be effectively treated by natural progesterone.

Progesterone (unlike estrogen and testosterone) is devoid of secondary sex characteristics. Thus its effects in promoting the development of the fetus are independent of the baby's gender. The fetus is allowed to develop according to its own DNA code and not be affected by the hormones of the mother.

Progesterone increases energy production (probably by helping the thyroid hormone work more efficiently), causing a slight rise in body temperature. This is called the *thermogenic* effect of progesterone and can be used to indicate ovulation for women who want to know when (and if) ovulation occurs.

The fall of progesterone levels at menopause is proportionately much greater than the fall of estrogen levels. While estrogen falls only 40 to 60 percent from baseline on average, the decline in progesterone levels is twelve times greater, according to endocrinologist Jerilynn Prior, M.D. Postmenopausal progesterone levels in some women are actually *lower* than those of males. This is an odd circumstance, considering the importance of progesterone as a precursor of all the steroid hormones. Furthermore, progesterone has many other important intrinsic functions that, one would think, need to be continued for good health. There is no reason to believe that postmenopausal women require less progesterone than men.

HOW PROGESTERONE AFFECTS THE BODY

Progesterone has many beneficial actions throughout the body. The list on page 72 provides an indication of its diversity and importance. Since progesterone protects against the undesirable side effects of unopposed estrogen, whether occurring from within the body as a result of anovulatory cycles or as a consequence of estrogen supplementation or exposure to xenoestrogens, these effects will be included in the list.

Estrogen allows the influx of water and sodium into cells, causing water retention and high blood pressure. Estrogen also reduces the amount of oxygen present in the cells, opposes the action of thyroid, promotes histamine release (which causes allergy-type symptoms), promotes blood clotting thus increasing the risk of stroke and embolism, thickens bile and promotes gallbladder disease, and causes copper retention and zinc loss. Estrogen unopposed by progesterone also decreases sex drive, increases the likelihood of fibrocystic breasts, uterine fibroids, uterine (endometrial) cancer, and breast cancer. All of these undesirable effects of estrogen are countered by progesterone. Restoring proper progesterone levels is what is known as restoring hormone *balance*.

PROGESTERONE AND STEROID SYNTHESIS

Before discussing the third important function of progesterone, its role in making steroid hormones, it may be helpful to review how cholesterol and pregnenolone are made. Cholesterol is made

Functions of Progesterone

- is a precursor of other sex hormones, including estrogen and testosterone
- maintains secretory endometrium (uterine lining)
- is necessary for the survival of the embryo and fetus throughout gestation
- protects against fibrocystic breasts
- is a natural diuretic
- helps use fat for energy
- functions as a natural antidepressant
- helps thyroid hormone action
- normalizes blood clotting
- restores sex drive
- helps normalize blood sugar levels
- normalizes zinc and copper levels
- restores proper cell oxygen levels
- has a thermogenic (temperature-raising) effect
- protects against endometrial cancer
- helps protect against breast cancer
- builds bone and is protective against osteoporosis
- is a precursor of cortisone synthesis by adrenal cortex

by cells throughout the body, particularly in the liver, from acetate (a small two-carbon compound), a substance derived in the breakdown of sugars and fats. There is a common myth that eating cholesterol causes cholesterol levels to rise, but the truth is that eating more sugar, starch, and any fat in excess of need can cause cholesterol levels to rise. Some 75 percent of our total cholesterol is made from these foods rather than from cholesterol intake per se. A rise in cholesterol levels has more to do with how much sugar, refined starch, and saturated fat we eat, whether we're getting enough fiber, vitamins, and minerals in our diets, how much we exercise, and what our stress levels are. Genetics also plays a large part in cholesterol levels.

The production of hormones is a dynamic, fluctuating system, constantly responding to changing body conditions and needs. Hormones are the control messengers for a vast, interrelated, ever-changing network of organ-system commands. As such, they must be continually synthesized for moment-to-moment situational needs and likewise must be metabolized and removed from the system when no longer needed in order for their presence to fall as their need diminishes. (The liver is constantly metabolizing and excreting hormones as they pass through in the bloodstream.) Progesterone, in addition to its own hormonal effects, is a main player in the creation of all these hormones. Various cells in key organs throughout the body use progesterone to create the other specific hormones as needed, specifically the adrenal corticosteroids, estrogen, and testosterone.

This precursor aspect of progesterone distinguishes it from many other hormones that are at a metabolic end point, meaning they are unable to be used further except to be broken down for excretion. The synthetic progestins now being heavily promoted in hormone replacement therapy have undergone molecular alterations at unusual positions. As these strange, not-found-in-nature molecules travel down the hormone pathways, they occupy progesterone receptor sites, create actions different from natural progesterone, cannot be used as precursors of other hormones (as progesterone can), and are difficult for the body to metabolize and excrete. These molecular alterations carry a heavy burden of potential undesirable side effects. This, however, does not seem to deter the marketing of them. Physicians who are the targets of heavy pharmaceutical advertising (and unaware that natural progesterone is available) tend to accede to marketing pressure.

Natural progesterone is needed for the appropriate and balanced supply of all the steroid hormones. To overcome present marketing practices and restore natural progesterone to its proper place in the practice of medicine will apparently require reeducation of its diverse and important role in health by patients and doctors alike.

PROGESTERONE AND THE BRAIN

Although progesterone is not a sex hormone per se in that its presence doesn't confer the attributes of maleness or femaleness, it is important to central nervous system (the brain and spinal cord) function as are other sex hormones. Progesterone is concentrated in brain cells to levels 20 times higher than that of blood serum levels. Such high concentrations in brain cells cannot be due to simple diffusion but require work on the part of brain cells. This alone strongly suggests that progesterone in brain cells must serve some important purpose.

Progesterone has long been known to have a calming or mildly sedating effect. This effect may be caused directly by progesterone, or it may be caused by substances created from progesterone that are active at GABA (gamma-aminobutyric acid) receptors. (GABA is an amino acid that acts as a neurotransmitter inhibitor and tends to have a calming effect.) Progesterone's sedation of the central nervous system is sufficiently potent in higher doses that it has been used as an anesthetic. When used in small doses, progesterone is commonly effective in restoring normal sleep patterns and promoting a sense of calm.

Even more intriguing and perhaps important to the practice of emergency medicine are recent studies on the effects of brain injury in rodents, which found that survival and recovery rates were higher in females than in males. However, when the male rodents were supplemented with progesterone, their survival and recovery from brain injuries paralleled that of female rodents. This benefit did not follow from estrogen supplementation. In fact, it is possible that estrogen supplementation has a deleterious effect on the brain. In a study of estrogen supplementation in a group of nurses, the data showed an *increase* in some types of strokes among the estrogen-using nurses. (Note that this result has not been widely publicized to doctors!) Unfortunately, none of the nurses in the study were being supplemented with progesterone, which might have prevented their strokes.

At this time, what we know about progesterone and the brain is that it is selectively concentrated in brain cells, has a calming effect, and has a beneficial effect on recovery from brain injury. And, as we shall see, progesterone has an important effect on libido or sex drive.

PROGESTERONE AND SEX DRIVE

The early proponents of estrogen replacement therapy (ERT) created a myth promising that estrogen would keep women "feminine" and sexually attractive "forever." Without the magic pill, they would turn into sexless hags and no longer be attractive to their husbands. It was a common misconception that older women were no longer interested in sex.

In my medical practice, many premenopausal women told me that in truth they were less interested in sex. Others, however, told me that as they approached menopause, they had become even more desirous of sex; it was their husbands whose sexual stamina was failing. The difference in the women, it seemed to me, related to whether or not the women were experiencing estrogen dominance, i.e., continued estrogen effects (monthly periods) without progesterone (anovulatory periods). The women losing interest in sex had water retention, fibrocystic breasts, depression, dry, wrinkling skin, and irregular, sometimes heavy periods. I gradually came to understand that these signs and symptoms were indicative of a progesterone deficiency caused by a failure to ovulate while estrogen continued to be produced, which is to say loss of sex drive correlates with progesterone deficiency, not estrogen deficiency. Women on estrogen replacement therapy coming to me for treatment of their osteoporosis also confided in me that they were unhappy with the fat accumulating at their hips and abdomen, their swollen breasts, and their loss of sex drive. Estrogen replacement had not restored their previous sex drive.

When these women used the progesterone cream supplementation I recommended, the story changed; they were delighted to report that their sex drive had returned. I received a Christmas card from one woman telling me that her bones were better, her skin was more youthful, and, by the way, her husband thanked me, too! I learned to ask my progesterone-using patients about their sex drives, and uniformly their eyes brightened and they told me their sex life was better after progesterone therapy than any time during the 10 to 15 years before menopause. Progesterone had restored normal sex drive.

My clinical experience with these patients was at odds with what I had learned in medical school. I had been taught that only estrogen and testosterone were vital to normal sex drive. Pharmacologic (abnormally large) doses of progesterone, when given to male rats and lizards, had been found to inhibit sexual behavior. But a 1994 study found that physiologic (much smaller) doses of progesterone had the opposite effect, i.e., it restored sex drive.

But what about females?

In another recent study, female hamsters with their ovaries removed did not show sexual behavior unless areas of their brains vital for sex drive were stimulated by progesterone. When stimulated with estrogen alone, these brain areas did not stimulate normal sexual activity. When progesterone was added, sexual activity revived.

While I grant that hamsters are not humans, it is clear that, in most female mammals, the rise and fall of sex hormones coordinates sexual behavior so that mating is most likely to occur near the time of ovulation. This, after all, is the primary function of sex drive. This study thus shows that sex drive is a function of both estrogen and progesterone, and probably also of testosterone. The administration of estrogen in the absence of progesterone does not accomplish stimulation of sex drive. (I would like to see a study where progesterone alone was administered!) In humans, estrogen production falls only 40 to 60 percent at menopause, whereas progesterone falls to close to zero when ovulation no longer occurs. This explains the loss of sex drive in my premenopausal patients with estrogen sufficient for monthly periods (and in postmenopausal women on ERT) but lacking in progesterone and the resumption of normal sex drive when progesterone was added.

Among many researchers, testosterone is given credit for being the hormone attached to sex drive in both males and females. It is widely assumed that the increased sex drive in fertile women at ovulation correlates with a timely spurt of testosterone. In a test of this hypothesis, Drs. Ben C. Campbell and Peter T. Ellison of Harvard University measured daily salivary testosterone levels among regularly cycling women and did find a very small peak, as expected. In an interesting aside, to verify that the women were in fact ovulating, they also checked midcycle progesterone levels. To their surprise, seven of the 18 women in the study (age range 24 to 42 years, average 29 years of age) did not ovulate, although they were menstruating. This is still further evidence that anovulatory cycles are common among relatively young, regularly cycling women in the United States.

It is important to be reminded again of the complex interplay and delicate balance of hormones in the human body and the difference between taking physiologic and pharmacologic doses of hormones. *Physiologic* (equivalent to normal body function) doses are meant to be replacement doses for a specific hormone deficiency. They are not meant to exceed normal bodily production and they promote no abnormal actions in the body. *Pharmacologic* (drug) doses, on the other hand, are considerably greater than normal production and lead not only to suppression of natural hormone production, but to actions different than those found with normal hormone levels. In the case of progesterone, pharmacologic doses may actually inhibit sex drive whereas physiologic doses stimulate sex drive. In my practice I recommended a progesterone cream that supplied only about 20 to 30 milligrams per day, simulating normal progesterone production. Many physicians, for reasons I do not understand, opt for doses 10 to 20 times higher. When they report that they do not see the resurgence of sex drive as I have found with my patients, it is not a surprise to me.

PROGESTERONE IN MEN

Progesterone is the precursor of testosterone and corticosteroids, meaning the body uses progesterone to make these other hormones. Progesterone in men is synthesized by their testes to produce testosterone and in their adrenals to produce corticosteroids. Progesterone levels in men are naturally much lower than in women during their fertile years. However, after menopause (or even 10 to 15 years before menopause), some women's progesterone levels fall below that of same-age men. Typically, healthy men continue to produce normal testosterone and corticosteroid levels into their seventies and eighties.

I recall reading in the *Medical Tribune* over fifteen years ago of a study involving progesterone supplementation in men. Progesterone given to college-age men resulted in no apparent change in general stamina, vigor, or sex drive. Testosterone levels fell, however, to levels low enough to inhibit sperm maturation. Since many testosterone receptors also accept progesterone (and with similar results), it is likely that a biofeedback mechanism in the brain reduces testosterone production when high levels of progesterone are present. Thus it appears that pharmacologic doses of progesterone in men act only as a contraceptive.

Among men with prostate cancer, it is common practice to castrate them either surgically or chemically to reduce their testosterone level as low as possible in the belief that this suppresses prostate cancer growth. The abrupt, almost total absence of testosterone creates a sort of male menopause, often complete with hot flashes. Disturbing as this is, it is perhaps more important that the lack of testosterone will bring on an acceleration of osteoporosis within just a year or so. Like progesterone, testosterone can stimulate new bone formation, increasing bone density, and a lack of it can cause osteoporosis.

Progesterone and testosterone are equivalent hormones in regard to new bone formation. They and the corticosteroids compete for the same osteoblast receptor sites on the bones, with testosterone and progesterone stimulating new bone formation whereas corticosteroids inhibit it. If one wishes to prevent or treat the castration-induced osteoporosis, it is possible to safely supplement progesterone to replace testosterone in these men. While my experience in using progesterone under these circumstances is limited, and insufficient for statistical evaluation, the results to date have been encouraging. Hopefully further research will emerge to better evaluate this potential benefit of progesterone.

Chapter 7

THE DRAMATIC DIFFERENCE BETWEEN PROGESTERONE AND PROGESTINS

Your physician probably believes that the synthetic progestins such as Provera (medroxyprogesterone acetate) are the same as natural progesterone. This is a common and very unfortunate misunderstanding. Most doctors don't have the time to keep up on the latest drug research, so they rely on pharmaceutical company ads or representatives for their information. The pharmaceutical companies have no interest in selling natural progesterone because they can't patent it, so they have no interest in sponsoring research or passing on information about it. Thus we have a widespread misconception among American doctors that natural progesterone has the same side effects as the progestins—an error that is dramatically affecting the health and well-being of millions of American women. In fact, natural progesterone used in physiologic doses (no greater than what the body normally should be making) has no known side effects, while the synthetic progestins have many.

There have been many, many excellent studies done on natural progesterone, which are referenced on page 342–343. A small but interesting study was done when Joel Hargrove et al. (1989) compared oral progesterone with Provera (medroxyprogesterone acetate). Both were combined with different forms of estrogen in menopausal women. The group on progesterone found symptomatic improvement of menopausal symptoms, improved cholesterol levels, the absence of menstruation without the typical progestin and estrogen-related problems of abnormal tissue growth in the uterus, and no side effects. All ten of the women taking progesterone and estradiol wished to continue their hormone treatment, while two of the five women using estrone and medroxyprogesterone acetate discontinued their treatment due to side effects.

A much larger study done in 1995 (the PEPI trial) examined the effects of sex hormones on cholesterol and HDL-cholesterol as well as their effects on the endometrium. This three-year, multicenter, randomized, double-blind, placebo-controlled (the gold standard of medical research), $22-million, federally funded trial found that estrogen taken alone "significantly increased the occurrence of severe hyperplasia" in those women with an intact uterus (hyperplasia is considered to be a step along the pathway to cancer) whereas estrogen with natural progesterone or medroxyprogesterone acetate (the progestin) completely protected women from this side effect. Estrogen caused these precancerous changes in one-third of the women who took estrogen alone. However, estrogen did effectively lower total cholesterol and raise HDL-cholesterol (the "good" cholesterol), followed closely by the estrogen/natural progesterone combination, which was significantly superior to the estrogen/progestin combination. In the news items that followed the publication of this study, natural progesterone was described as "a little known 'natural' form of progesterone derived from wild yams or soybeans." From my point of view, the trial would have been even better had they included a subgroup of women using only natural progesterone.

While I get phone calls every day from health professionals around the world who are using progesterone with great success, we are very much in need of further clinical trials comparing progesterone therapy alone with progesterone/estrogen therapy. Since the menopausal decrease of estrogen is only 40 to 60 percent, true estrogen deficiency is a misnomer. My experience, and the experience of many of the doctors who correspond with or call me, has been that most menopausal symptoms will respond to progesterone supplementation alone. If they do not, such women may need very low-dose estrogen supplementation for several years, which can then be gradually discontinued without recurrence of the symptoms.

THE DIFFERENCE BETWEEN SYNTHETIC DRUGS AND NATURAL COMPOUNDS

A synthetic drug is man-made and usually not found in nature by itself. (If you want to be very technical, the natural progesterone derived from wild yam or soybeans could be called semisynthetic, because although it is identical to the molecule found in the human body it does not come directly from the human body, but is formulated from a plant source [diosgenin] in a laboratory.) Aspirin is an example of another drug originally made from a natural substance. It has its medicinal origins in trees of the *salix* species, most commonly known as willow and poplar. Various teas, decoctions, tinctures, and poultices of *salix* were used medicinally in America, Europe, and Asia for centuries to relieve pain, especially the pain of headaches and arthritis.

In the late 1800s laws were passed in the United States that allowed medicines to be patented only if they were *not* natural substances. If a drug company discovered a naturally occurring medicine, anyone else was free to capitalize on the discovery. Needless to say, drug companies quickly became disinterested in naturally occurring medicines. These days, when a plant with medicinal value is discovered, the "active ingredient" is isolated and transformed. This new molecule can be patented. In the case of *salix,* a chemist at the Bayer company in Germany synthesized acetylsalicyclic acid in 1897 and aspirin was born.

While there is no doubt that aspirin is a wonderful drug—Americans consume somewhere around 30 billion tablets every year—willow bark does not have aspirin's side effects. Aspirin and the whole family of nonsteroidal anti-inflammatory pain relievers (NSAIDs) have a wide range of side effects, mostly in the area of stomach inflammation, and cause in excess of 6,000 fatalities and 30,000 hospitalizations every year due to bleeding in the stomach or intestines. Acetaminophen (e.g., Tylenol) is damaging to the liver. Aspirin and acetaminophen, however, are readily available and easy to use—willow bark is neither.

The history of creating synthetic drugs consistently shows that separating the so-called active ingredient from the rest of the plant to create substances not found in nature almost always creates harmful side effects, whereas plant medicines, used properly, rarely have harmful side effects. Nature has a great wisdom that humans have not been able to duplicate in synthetic drugs. Over millions of years of evolution, our biochemistry has become integrated very specifically with the natural world. Our bodies know how to take natural substances, use them for energy, maintenance, and repair, and then efficiently excrete them when they are used up. Conversely, when synthetic, chemically altered hormone drugs occupy cell receptors, the message they convey may be different, even contrary to the hormone they are meant to simulate. Such effects are called side effects. Further, being foreign to normal metabolic processes, they cannot be excreted as well.

Tryptophan, a naturally occurring amino acid found in the greatest abundance in milk and turkey, became very popular some twenty years ago as a sleep remedy and antidepressant. It is very effective and has minimal side effects when used sensibly. A contaminated batch of tryptophan from Japan killed a number of people and caused a debilitating disease in others, so the FDA asked manufacturers for a voluntary recall of the substance as a supplement, meaning it is effectively banned in the United States. Ironically, however, tryptophan is still used in the United States in baby formulas and tube feedings for the elderly. If it wasn't present it wouldn't be nutritionally complete! There is not a shred of evidence anywhere that *uncontaminated* tryptophan taken in prescribed doses is harmful. Coincindentally—or perhaps not so coincidentally—the pharmaceutical industry has recently poured millions into advertising and public relations to introduce a new class of antidepressant prescription drugs, including Prozac, that work in a way similar to tryptophan. These drugs differ only slightly in their action from tryptophan and other naturally occurring amino acids but differ greatly in their risk of side effects. Prozac alone has been directly linked to over 1000 deaths in the few short years it has been on the market and yet, being accepted by the FDA, enjoys phenomenal sales.

Many synthetic drugs are made patentable simply by changing a few atoms of the natural substance. This may sound harmless enough, but the addition or subtraction of a few atoms of a molecule can make a big difference in their effects on the body. This holds especially true with hormones. Tiny amounts can create major effects on the body. For example, the molecular difference between testosterone and estradiol (a form of estrogen) is one hydrogen atom and a couple of double bonds. Amazing! Adding or subtracting one hydrogen atom at a specific place on a molecule can make the difference between a man and a woman!

Now compare that exquisite level of biochemical specificity to what a pharmaceutical company does to a perfectly good natural hormone—they add whole chains of molecules! They do this not to make a better drug, but to make one that behaves similarly yet is different enough to be patentable.

I am reminded of a menopausal woman in Canada who sent me a ten-pound packet of her medical records from the five or six doctors she had consulted, asking for my advice. In the packet was a series of laboratory tests for serum progesterone. The patient had been put on the progestin, medroxyprogesterone acetate (Provera), and her doctor had ordered a serum progesterone level. Finding it still zero, he doubled the progestin dose and ordered a second test. This, too, was zero. He doubled the progestin dose again and ordered a third test, which again indicated zero progesterone. But on this lab report the technician had written, "Doctor, you are giving this woman Provera. You are ordering tests for serum progesterone. Provera is not progesterone!" By this time, the patient was experiencing numerous side effects from the drug, specifically loss of appetite, nausea, indigestion, fatigue, and depression. I circled the lab tech's comment in red and sent it back to the woman with an information sheet on natural progesterone. Several months later I got a very nice note from her telling me how much better she felt using natural progesterone and that she had fired all but one of her doctors.

WHAT IS A PROGESTIN?

A progestin is often defined as "any compound able to sustain the human secretory endometrium." This refers to the ability to keep the lining of the uterus healthy and blood-rich in preparation for pregnancy and to support the developing embryo. When a woman comes to the end of her monthly cycle and no pregnancy has occurred, the levels of her reproductive hormones drop dramatically and in response the lining of the uterus is shed in menstruation.

Throughout much of the medical literature, natural progesterone is either equated with progestins, as if they were the same thing, or classed as one of the progestins, which, strictly speaking, is also incorrect. There is only one *progesterone,* the specific molecule made by the adrenal glands or by the ovary as a consequence of ovulation. (To complicate things even further, European writers refer to progestins as gestagens or progestogens.) I would define progestins as any compound *other than natural progesterone* able to sustain the human secretory endometrium.

Why do I insist on this separation? First and foremost, natural progesterone is necessary for the survival and development of the embryo and throughout pregnancy. On the other hand, Provera, the most commonly prescribed progestin, carries the warning that its use in early pregnancy may *increase* the risk of early abortion or congenital deformities of the fetus. These are only two of the many serious side effects of the progestins. To appreciate the scope of progestin side effects, it is instructive to review the *Physicians' Desk Reference (PDR)* pages for medroxyprogesterone acetate. An *abbreviated* list from the 1995 *Physicians' Desk Reference (PDR)* follows:

POTENTIAL SIDE EFFECTS OF
MEDROXYPROGESTERONE ACETATE (PROVERA)

Warnings:
- Increased risk of birth defects such as heart and limb defects if taken during the first four months of pregnancy.
- Beagle dogs given this drug developed malignant mammary nodules.
- Discontinue this drug if there is sudden or partial loss of vision.

- This drug passes into breast milk, consequences unknown.
- May contribute to thrombophlebitis, pulmonary embolism, and cerebral thrombosis.

Contraindications:

Thrombophlebitis, thromboembolic disorders, cerebral apoplexy; liver dysfunction or disease; known or suspected malignancy of breast or genital organs; undiagnosed vaginal bleeding; missed abortion; or known sensitivity.

Precautions:
- May cause fluid retention, epilepsy, migraine, asthma, cardiac or renal dysfunction.
- May cause breakthrough bleeding or menstrual irregularities.
- May cause or contribute to depression.
- The effect of prolonged use of this drug on pituitary, ovarian, adrenal, hepatic, or uterine function is unknown.
- May decrease glucose tolerance; diabetic patients must be carefully monitored.
- May increase the thrombotic disorders associated with estrogens.

Adverse Reactions:
- May cause breast tenderness and galactorrhea.
- May cause sensitivity reactions such as urticaria, pruritus, edema, or rash.
- May cause acne, alopecia, and hirsutism.
- Edema, weight changes (increase or decrease).
- Cervical erosions and changes in cervical secretions.
- Cholestatic jaundice.
- Mental depression, pyrexia, nausea, insomnia, or somnolence.

- Anaphylactoid reactions and anaphylaxis (severe acute allergic reactions).
- Thrombophlebitis and pulmonary embolism.
- Breakthrough bleeding, spotting, amenorrhea, or changes in menses.

When taken with estrogens, the following have been observed:
- Rise in blood pressure, headache, dizziness, nervousness, fatigue.
- Changes in sex drive, hirsutism and loss of scalp hair, decrease in T3 uptake values.
- Premenstrual-like syndrome, changes in appetite.
- Cystitis-like syndrome (urinary tract infections).
- Erythema multiforme, erythema nodosum, hemorrhagic eruption, itching.

Most of the progestins are synthesized from progesterone or from another hormone called nortestosterone and are not found in any living forms. They may be only a couple of atoms different from natural progesterone, but it is evident that such a seemingly slight shift can make the difference between a successful pregnancy and an unsuccessful one.

Because progesterone is a natural hormone, the body is normally able to produce it, use it, and eliminate it as needed. The synthetic progestins, on the other hand, are not well processed by the body. Their activity is prolonged, creating reactions in the body that are not consistent with natural progesterone.

Progestins bind to the same receptors in the cell as progesterone, but from that point on they carry different messages to the cell. In other words, the parts of the body that need progesterone at first identify progestins as a progesterone. However, the small alterations in the progestins will then convey a different message. This undoubtedly explains the alarming array of listed warnings, contraindications, precautions, and adverse reactions to progestins, all of which are uncharacteristic of natural progesterone. To complicate matters even more, synthetic progestins generally bind to the progesterone receptor more tenaciously and thereby inhibit the action of the natural hormone. Furthermore, each variety of progestin differs from the others and carries its own unique array of side effects.

Progestins in general are similar to progesterone and estrogen in their ability to be easily absorbed into the body through the skin (transdermally). Thus some hormone replacement therapies utilize a patch that gradually releases the hormones into the body. If natural progesterone is taken orally, it is transported to the liver first, where a majority is eliminated in bile, a substance made by the liver. Natural hormones are used and eliminated more quickly than the synthetic versions.

Progestins and estrogen cause water retention, often accompanied by hypertension (high blood pressure). Natural progesterone helps balance fluid in the cells and appears to have a protective effect *against* hypertension. While progesterone has a beneficial effect of improving the ability of the body to use and eliminate fats, progestins have the opposite effect. As described in the PEPI study, the combination of estrogen and progesterone was clearly superior to estrogen and Provera in its cholesterol effects. Progestins share with natural progesterone the ability to promote new bone formation but with less success. Dr. Jerilynn Prior has found a 5-percent increase in bone mineral density using medroxyprogesterone acetate (Provera) in postmenopausal osteoporotic patients. In my experience, the typical bone mineral density increase shown with natural progesterone was 15 percent.

The following chart indicates some of the differences between natural progesterone and the synthetic progestins:

Conditions	Natural Progesterone	Progestin
sodium and water into body cells		√
loss of mineral electrolytes from cells		√
intracellular edema		√
depression		√
birth defect risks		√
more body hair, thinner scalp hair		√
thrombophlebitis, embolism risk		√
decreased glucose tolerance		√
allergic reactions		√
cholestatic jaundice risk		√
acne, skin rashes		√
protects against endometrial cancer	√	√
protects against breast cancer	√	
normalizes libido	√	
less hirsutism, regrowth of scalp hair	√	
improves lipid profile	√	
improves in vitro fertilization	√	
improves new bone formation	√	modestly
improves sleep patterns	√	

Table 1: Comparison of the effects of natural progesterone and synthetic progestins.

PROGESTINS GAVE BIRTH TO THE SEXUAL REVOLUTION

Given all that is known about the great difference of actions and of safety between progesterone and the synthetic progestins, why is it that progestins dominate in the role of progesterone supplementation? Aside from the obvious financial gains to be made from a patentable molecule, the answer lies in their use in contraceptive pills.

Until the late 1960s, there were two main factors holding back the sexual revolution: the fear of unwanted pregnancy and venereal disease. In industrialized Western culture, the development of the automobile effectively removed the young from their usual adult chaperones. Then the advent of penicillin and the apparent easy cures of gonorrhea and syphilis removed the perceived threat of venereal disease. All that was needed for the explosion of the sexual revolution was a convenient, effective (and private) contraceptive. Thus the stage was set for progestational drugs.

When progesterone became obtainable (from plant sources) in sufficient amounts for aggressive research by private biochemical industries, it did not take long for the development of oral, highly effective (for birth control), synthetic progestins.

But how does a hormone that is crucial to the survival and development of the embryo in pregnancy act as a birth control pill? During each monthly cycle, eggs mature in both ovaries until ovulation occurs in one of them, creating the corpus luteum, which is responsible for a great surge of progesterone production. This surge of progesterone, as one of its effects, stops ovulation in the other ovary (which is why fraternal twins are born only once for every 300 pregnancies). If sufficient progesterone is provided prior to ovulation, neither ovary produces an egg. This inhibition of ovulation was the original mechanism of action of progestin contraception.

The advantages of progestins were: (1) ease of delivery system [oral tablets], (2) consistent potency [guaranteed contraception], (3) they lasted longer in the body [inability of the body to metabolize them], and (4) a patentable [i.e., profitable] product. In those days natural progesterone supplementation required expensive, painful injections or rectal or vaginal suppositories.

The long lists of undesirable and potentially serious side effects from progestins are dutifully printed in the *PDR* and in product information sheets, usually in type so small that only the most curious would read them. No one really wanted to know of them because of what was being offered: sex without fear of pregnancy.

Then another use was found for the progestins. As physicians began using estrogen therapy for menopausal symptoms, problems arose. During the 1970s it became obvious that postmenopausal women taking estrogen alone for menopausal symptoms had an increased risk of endometrial cancer. This cancer rarely if ever occurred during one's fertile years when normal levels of estrogen and progesterone were present. Testing of postmenopausal women with combined hormone therapy (using both estrogen and a progestin) found that estrogen-induced endometrial cancer could be largely prevented. In the midseventies, a Mayo Clinic consensus conference concluded that estrogen should never be given to any woman with an intact uterus (any woman who hasn't had a hysterectomy) without also giving progesterone or a progestin as protection from endometrial cancer. The effect of this was to expand the market for progestins to include *all* women, whether menstruating or postmenopausal! The financial implications of this are difficult to exaggerate.

Even the threat of breast cancer has not stopped the market for estrogen/progestin hormone therapy. A 1989 report by Leif Bergkvist et al. convincingly showed that supplemental estrogen (at least estradiol) when combined with a progestin "seems to be associated with a slightly *increased* risk of breast cancer, which is not prevented and may even be *increased* by the addition of the progestins" (emphasis added). This has not slowed the progestin bandwagon. Meanwhile, natural progesterone, as we shall see in a later chapter, can help *prevent* breast cancer.

Women should be upset that the hormone "balancing" being done to them uses synthetic and abnormal versions of the real goods, when the natural hormones are available, safer, and more appropriate to their bodies.

Are progestins the wave of the future? We should hope not. Our goal should be that when hormone therapy is indicated, the hormones should be the natural ones used in physiologic dosages. It can be taken as a rule that, among steroids, any unnatural changes in their molecular makeup will alter their effects. It should be clear that nature produces the substances that serve us best.

Chapter 8

SEX HORMONES AND THE BRAIN

We're all familiar with jokes about people—males and females—whose brains appear to be located below the waist instead of in their heads. In truth, brain function involves the whole body, as we shall see. The main operating systems are indeed in the head, and the sex hormones play important roles there, too.

THE BASICS OF BRAIN COMMUNICATION

Weighing only three pounds, the brain is composed of eight billion nerve cells held in specific structural arrangements by filaments, as well as by smaller, specialized connective tissue cells called glial cells, which comprise half of the brain's weight. Each adult brain nerve cell has on average 5000 extensions, called synapses, by which it communicates with other brain cells. That means the brain has eight billion times 5000, or 4×10^{13} connections, a number almost too large to comprehend. If we think of the brain as a computer, that number of connections is many times larger than that found in the world's largest computer.

Among mammals, brain size is less important than function. An adult elephant's brain is four times larger and a whale's seven times larger than a human's, yet their mental ability is less than an orangutan's, whose brain is only one-third as large as a human's. The number of interconnections plus the range of sensitivity and complexity make the human brain a wonder to behold.

Brain cells communicate with each other via electrochemical impulses carried between the synapses by neurotransmitters, which are substances made up of amino acids. The brain communicates with all tissues and cells of the body via neurotransmitters circulating in the bloodstream and generated by nerve extensions throughout the body.

When carried any distance, nerves are sheathed in an off-white insulating covering called myelin, which protects the nerves from trauma and chemical erosion and prevents short-circuiting of the electric impulse along the way. All along the peripheral nerves (throughout the body) are special cells called Schwann cells, which continually maintain the myelin sheath. If the myelin sheath becomes eroded for any reason, nerve function is adversely effected. This is known as peripheral neuropathy, such as occurs in diabetic neuropathy, Guillain-Barré syndrome, and multiple sclerosis, for example.

Guess what the ability of the Schwann cell to perform this vital function is a result of? Right—progesterone! In fact, the Schwann cell itself makes progesterone for this function. Recent research shows that anything that interferes with progesterone receptors (e.g., the "morning after" birth control pill, RU-486) in Schwann cells stops the production of protective myelin.

Within the brain, nerve cells in one part of the brain communicate with nerve cells in other parts of the brain and these nerves also need to be protected with myelin sheaths. It is not yet known, but it is likely that here, too, progesterone is needed.

Brain cells communicate with the body in other ways, too. Some brain cells make special neurotransmitters that flow through minute veins to the pituitary to tell the pituitary to make hormones that affect various organs of the body, such as the ovaries, testes, adrenal gland, and thyroid gland. Minute amounts of neurotransmitters also flow through the bloodstream and to the receptors present in all tissues, including white blood cells. The brain is in touch with every part of our body at all times. Not only does the brain tell the body what to do, but it monitors the response (electrolyte balance, hormone production, oxygen levels, nutrients, inflammation, temperature, blood pressure, and so on) to determine what to do next, even during sleep. This is the biofeedback cycle essential for maintaining our optimum health. The sex hormones are major players in this ongoing cycle.

HOW THE INNER AND OUTER BRAINS REGULATE THE BODY

We have one brain inside another, and they are different from each other. The outer layer of the brain, which we see in pictures of whole brains, is called the *cortex*. Deep inside the brain, however, is another area of cortex called the *limbic brain*.

Both the outer and inner areas of the brain are subject to learning and conditioning, both require optimal nutrition for best performance, and the sex hormones are important in both.

The outer brain is the one we are conscious of. By means of the outer brain cortex we receive our senses of sight, hearing, and touch; we control our speech, our muscular movements, and voluntary behavior; we make our plans, ponder the future, and grapple with language, grocery bills, mathematics, other symbolic thinking, and much, much more. Different sites within the outer cortex correlate with specific functions that are more or less independent of each other. A lesion in the sight area does not affect our hearing, for example.

The inner, limbic brain is the seat of emotions, our sense of pain, our primary drives (fight, flight, feeding, and sex), involuntary reactions, and all the automatic adjustments necessary for body function, including the immune system. Whereas the outer cortex functions are separated into different anatomical sites, the limbic brain is more interrelated in the sense that all its different functions affect each other. For example, if something frightens us, our pupils will dilate, our mouth goes dry, our muscles tense, blood is diverted away from our stomach and to our muscles, our skin color pales, and we may urinate or defecate involuntarily. Our reaction to stress is a limbic brain function.

As we've already seen, the menstrual cycle occurs as the result of a feedback loop of coordinated messages from the hypothalamus (in the limbic brain), to the pituitary gland, to the ovaries, and back to the hypothalamus. Thus it is natural that stress can affect one's menstrual cycles, too. It is wise therefore to always keep in mind that menstrual irregularity may arise simply from stress.

ESTROGEN AND THE BRAIN

It is the experience of many women that menopause is associated with some depression and that estrogen supplementation can lift one's mood. There is a good explanation for this. Elevated mood occurs when noradrenalin, the form of adrenaline active in brain cells, is raised. This happens, for example, after fairly strenuous exercise or when some pleasant excitement happens. Noradrenalin is inactivated by the enzyme monoamine oxidase (MAO). If, for some reason, MAO is relatively high compared to noradrenalin production, a depressed mood results. Estrogen inhibits MAO and thus raises the mood. (Synthetic progestins, on the other hand, tend to stimulate MAO and thus can lead to a depressed mood.)

Long-term use of estrogen, however, can have a negative effect on mood. This has to do with copper and zinc ratios. Copper and zinc are important cofactors for brain enzymes. Estrogen increases a blood protein, ceruloplasmin, which binds to copper and prevents dietary copper from finding its way into brain cells. Too much ceruloplasmin leaves too much copper in the blood, causing zinc levels to drop in the blood and the brain. The result is an imbalance that leads to exaggerated stress reactions, serious mood swings, and depression. (Sounds like PMS, doesn't it?)

Estrogen has several other effects that can adversely affect the brain. Estrogen tends to make blood more likely to clot. In the Nurses' Questionnaire Study, for example, the relative risk of ischemic stroke (blockage of blood vessels by clots) mortality among estrogen users compared to non-estrogen-using nurses was 46 percent greater after adjustment for age and other risk factors. That is, the risk of dying from an ischemic (more generally called thromboembolic) stroke was 46 percent higher among the estrogen-using nurses.

As a compensatory effect for its increased clotting risk, estrogen promotes blood vessel dilation. This, along with estrogen's water retention effect, explains why estrogen can induce migraine headaches in women. Cyclical migraine attacks (usually just preceding menstruation) are classic symptoms of estrogen dominance. Fortunately, progesterone promotes normal vascular tone and thus can prevent migraine. Again, hormone balance is the key.

Estrogen also tends to suppress thyroid gland function. Women who have estrogen dominance are often diagnosed with hypothyroidism despite normal levels of T3 and T4. The metabolic rate of all cells is dependent on thyroid hormone function, and brain cells are no exception. The impact of low thyroid on the brain is multidimensional.

One of the major brain neurotransmitters is a substance known as GABA (gamma-aminobutyric acid), the function of which is to "tune down" cell excitability. The production of GABA is related to cell metabolism; the lower the metabolic rate, the less GABA is formed. When estrogen interferes with thyroid production and slows the metabolism of brain cells, it indirectly decreases GABA production and increases brain cell excitability, a factor in epilepsy.

Further, the respiratory enzymes of cells are thyroid-dependent. When thyroid function is low, cellular oxygen is low (cellular hypoxia). Thus estrogen-induced thyroid interference contributes to less-than-optimal brain function. Cell oxygen is, fortunately, enhanced by vitamin E and progesterone. This is probably the primary explanation for the increased mental acuity in many elderly women with signs of senility when they begin using progesterone.

The makers of HRT have reported claims of sharper brain function in older women receiving hormone replacement therapy (HRT), and the presumption was made that this was due to estrogen. The more likely reason is that the women seeking HRT were of a higher socioeconomic class with better diets, more years of education, and more favorable access to medical care, with a greater likelihood of having received thyroid supplements and vitamin E than the control group.

Finally, a complete lack of estrogen appears to have no deleterious effect on brain function. Recall that hormones work only if cells have receptors for them. A recent tragic case involved a 28-year-old man with a genetic mutation such that he completely lacked estrogen receptors. (Men also make estrogen.) In this case, tests of brain function showed no abnormality, despite the complete absence of estrogen effect.

PROGESTERONE AND THE BRAIN

Progesterone, like other fat-soluble compounds, is found in brain cells. What is surprising is that its concentration in brain cells is 20 times higher than blood serum levels. The same is true of testosterone and DHEA. It is fair, I believe, to infer that brain cells do this for a purpose. Let's look at some of the evidence for progesterone's effect in the brain.

PROGESTERONE AND FETAL BRAIN DEVELOPMENT

Progesterone appears to play a critical role in fetal brain development. During pregnancy, placental production of progesterone increases from 20 milligrams a day to over 350 milligrams a day during the last trimester. This is a phenomenal level of hormone. Progesterone promotes metabolism of maternal fat for energy and maintains stable blood glucose, both of which support fetal growth and development, especially of the brain. The brain requires approximately three times more energy than other body tissues. The brain of neonates is proportionately much larger relative to the body than it is in adults. Thus energy requirements for the brain of a neonate are especially crucial.

In this regard, Dr. Katherina Dalton has reported that babies of mothers who received natural progesterone showed greatly improved intelligence. Ray Peat, Ph.D., in his book *Progesterone in Orthomolecular Medicine,* published in 1993, reports, "Other investigators find that progesterone babies have strong, serene, independent characters." It is quite likely that, in addition to the improved cellular energy and stable glucose levels, progesterone has specific beneficial effects on brain cell maturation through mechanisms yet unknown. This in itself is not surprising. Spina bifida (incomplete closure of the lower end of the spinal cord) can be largely prevented by small but adequate doses of folic acid, and the mechanism of action is also unknown at this time.

PROGESTERONE AND BRAIN INJURIES

Progesterone can reduce the severity of brain injuries. In an experiment by Robin Roof and her colleagues, deliberate laboratory-induced head trauma to rodents resulted in reduced mortality and more rapid recovery of function among females compared to males. When male animals were given estrogen, no survival or recovery advantage was found. In fact, postmortem examinations revealed that cerebral (brain) contusions and edema were killing neurons far beyond the site of the original injury. When male animals were given progesterone, however, their survival and recovery rates corresponded to that of female rats. Even though rats are not necessarily the same as humans, if I suffered a head injury and was lying in a coma, I hope someone would give me a good dose of natural progesterone.

PROGESTERONE AND THE ELDERLY

"Doctor, I can think again!" I have heard this so often from patients after they have started progesterone therapy that I now regard it as routine. A writer got back to the book she was writing. Another woman resumed her painting. Others are just happy to be able to deal with letter-writing and checkbook-balancing. When progesterone is supplemented in anovulatory premenopausal or postmenopausal women, mental clarity and concentration ("focusing") improves. Many families have told me of elderly female relatives languishing in nursing homes. After progesterone therapy is started, the family reports being surprised at the improved mental clarity and attitudes they observed. I was paid a visit by Dr. George Moraes, a gerontologist from São Paulo, Brazil. He told me of his ninety-one-year-old mother, who had been consigned to a nursing home because of weakness and senility. After Dr. Moraes had given her progesterone cream for her dry, fragile skin and osteoporosis, he was surprised on his next visit to see her improved cognitive, conversational, and socializing abilities—skills that had deteriorated in the preceding years.

Obviously, more research is needed. It would be interesting to test progesterone and other hormone (estrogen, testosterone, cortisol, and DHEA) levels in women with and without Alzheimer's disease. Since estrogen dominance and early follicle failure are common in the United States, it is tempting to speculate that progesterone deficiency is a factor in premature brain deterioration.

PROGESTERONE AND LIBIDO

Libido, or sex drive, though mediated by sex hormones, is really a brain function. Specific areas of the brain have been identified in mice, rats, and hamsters as essential for sexual receptivity and mounting behavior. When one or another of these areas is experimentally destroyed, sexual behavior is lost, regardless of hormone levels. In female hamsters with their ovaries removed, estrogen alone is insufficient to restore sexual receptivity; progesterone is required. The inference is that low doses of estrogen "prime" the brain cells but progesterone "turns on" the sex drive.

In male rats, pharmacologic (large) dosages of progesterone inhibit sexual behavior but physiologic (similar to what the body would naturally produce) doses appear to have an opposite effect, stimulating male copulatory behavior. Here we learn that a hormone usually considered to be a female hormone also works in males.

Admittedly, rats and hamsters are not human, and human sexuality is modified by numerous social, behavioral, and other factors. However, the underlying primary sexual drive in all mammals surely emanates from brain centers mediated by sex hormones. The effect of progesterone on human libido has been largely ignored in mainstream medical research. The common "wisdom" is that estrogen is the primary sex drive hormone in women. The experience of my progesterone patients, however, does not bear this out. Their flagging libido returned only when progesterone was added. Many of my medical colleagues have the notion that testosterone turns on libido in females, completely overlooking the role of progesterone.

POSTPARTUM BLUES

Many women experience depression in the days (and weeks) following childbirth. Other symptoms include headache, irritability, and sleeplessness. The depression can be incapacitating and prolonged. Research by Brian Harris and colleagues in Wales found that, among 120 women, those with the highest prenatal and lowest postnatal progesterone levels also scored highest on measures of postpartum depression scores.

Recall that as pregnancy advances, placental production of progesterone rises to levels of 350 to 400 milligrams a day, and the ovaries' contribution at that point is nil. With delivery, the placenta-derived progesterone is suddenly gone. The only source of progesterone at that time would be the adrenal glands. It is possible that adrenal exhaustion plays a role in a woman's inability to provide even a modicum of progesterone in the days following childbirth. Postpartum depression is notoriously difficult to treat. It would seem appropriate to measure progesterone levels a day or two after childbirth and, if found to be low, progesterone could be promptly supplemented. It is possible that this simple and safe therapy could make postpartum depression much easier to treat.

PROGESTERONE AND SLEEP PATTERNS

Eric Bravermen, M.D., reported (in *Total Health,* August 1993) the multiple benefits of natural progesterone and its superiority over synthetic progestins with their many deleterious side effects. In his review, Dr. Bravermen reported only one side effect of progesterone—increased (or a return to normal) sleepiness—which, as he described, is generally a beneficial side effect.

Many of my patients have volunteered that the first benefit they perceived from using natural progesterone was an improved sleep pattern. After years of unsettled sleep they now look forward to retiring each night because they know they will enjoy sound sleep and awake refreshed in the morning. This is one of the reasons I tend to recommend that progesterone cream be applied at bedtime.

Research concerning progesterone's role in brain cell function is still in its infancy. It is likely that as research progresses more discoveries of progesterone's benefits will emerge.

Chapter 9

HORMONE BALANCE AND THE MENSTRUAL CYCLE

The human menstrual cycle has been the subject of scientific investigation since the 1890s. The word *menstrual* comes from the Greek word for "month," which itself was derived from earlier roots meaning "moon," or the period of time of the waxing and waning of one new moon to the next. Despite a century of study, full understanding of the menstrual cycle eludes us. The workings of nature surpass our current levels of understanding.

Let's briefly review the menstrual cycle again. The hallmark of menstruation is the monthly vaginal flow of blood. From puberty to menopause, the female uterus prepares a specially thickened and blood-filled lining in preparation for a possible pregnancy. This lining is shed if fertilization of the egg does not occur in a timely fashion, and the preparation of the lining begins anew. The cycle of uterine preparation and shedding occurs at approximately monthly intervals. We know that this uterine cycle is under the control of ovarian-secreted hormones, namely estrogen and progesterone.

Estrogen dominates the first week or so after menstruation, starting the endometrial buildup as the ovarian follicles (the sacs that hold and mature the eggs) are stimulated to begin the development of an egg. In addition, estrogen causes an increase in vaginal mucus, making it more tolerant of male penetration during sexual activity, as well as increased secretion of the glands of the cervix, making it more hospitable to sperm.

About twelve days after the beginning of the previous menses, the rising estrogen (primarily estradiol) level peaks and then tapers off just as the follicle matures and just before ovulation. When the egg has been released from the follicle, the follicle then becomes the corpus luteum ("yellow body" in Latin), so named because the follicle that produced the egg appears as a small yellow body on the surface of the ovary. The corpus luteum is the site of progesterone production, which dominates the second half of the menstrual month, reaching a peak of about 20 milligrams per day. Progesterone production during the luteal phase of the cycle (days 12 to 26 of the menstrual cycle) leads to the maturing or ripening phase of the development of the thickened and blood-filled uterine lining, called the secretory endometrium, in anticipation of a possible fertilized egg. In addition, progesterone influences the cervical glands, causing the secretions to change from watery to sticky, much like an uncooked egg white. (Allowing cervical mucus to dry on a glass slide will allow the appearance of a "ferning" pattern during progesterone dominance, which is not seen during the time of estrogen dominance.)

The rise of progesterone at the time of ovulation also causes a rise in body temperature of about one degree Fahrenheit, a finding often used to indicate ovulation. If pregnancy does not occur within 10 to 15 days after ovulation, estrogen and progesterone levels fall abruptly, triggering the shedding of the accumulated secretory endometrium and the menstrual flow of blood. If pregnancy occurs, progesterone production increases, and this shedding of endometrium is prevented, thus preserving the developing embryo. As pregnancy progresses, progesterone production is taken over by the placenta, and its secretion gradually increases to levels of 300 to 400 milligrams per day during the third trimester.

THE RISE AND FALL OF HORMONE LEVELS

Thus the monthly rise and fall of estrogen and progesterone levels explain the events of menstruation. But what determines the synchronous cycling of these two hormones? The answer is found in two hormones secreted by the anterior pituitary gland in the brain: the gonadotropic hormone follicle-stimulating hormone (FSH) and luteinizing hormone (LH). Simply put, FSH drives the ovary to make estrogen, promotes maturation of the follicle, and, at the same time, sensitizes the follicle receptors to LH. Meanwhile, LH rises a day or two before ovulation, triggering ovulation, and then falls dramatically as the corpus luteum starts turning out progesterone.

Now the question becomes: What determines the marvelous synchrony of FSH and LH? The answer lies in the hypothalamus within the limbic brain, a primitive but remarkably complex and sensitive control system. The hypothalamus is situated immediately above the pituitary, where it monitors not only the levels of estrogen and progesterone, but also the various body effects they are creating and, with exquisite timing, produces and sends to the pituitary (via special veinlike channels) a hormone made of ten linked amino acids called gonadotropin-releasing hormone (GnRH), which is responsible for the release of either or both of the gonadotropins, FSH and LH. At the present, it is not known how a single hypothalamic hormone can control both FSH and LH.

The reproductive hormone cycle described above is pictured in the figure below.

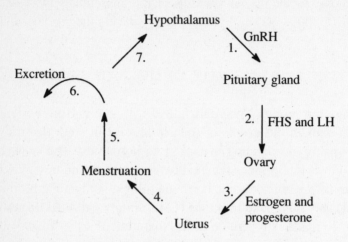

Figure 6:

1. *Low levels of estrogen and progesterone stimulate the hypothalamus to send* gonadotropin-releasing hormone *(GnRH) to the pituitary.*

2. *Stimulated by GnRH, the pituitary sends* follicle-stimulating hormone *(FSH) to the ovary, which initiates the maturation of ova in follicles and the production of estrogen. In about 10 days, the high estrogen level signals the pituitary production of* luteinizing hormone *(LH), which promotes ovulation.*

3. *The maturing ovarian follicles produce* estrogen, *which promotes proliferation of endometrial cells. After ovulation, the follicle (now the corpus luteum) produces* progesterone, *which becomes the dominant gonadal hormone during the second half of the cycle and converts the proliferative endometrium into the secretory endometrium.*

4. *If pregnancy does not occur, the corpus luteum involutes and the production of both estrogen and progesterone falls, a signal for the shedding of the endometrium, i.e., menstruation.*

5, 6. *Serum levels of estrogen and progesterone fall as they are metabolized and excreted from the body via the liver (bile) and urine.*

7. *The fall of estrogen and progesterone is detected by the hypothalamus, which then initiates another round of GnRH, starting another cycle.*

Another illustration of the hormone changes during a normal menstrual cycle is depicted below:

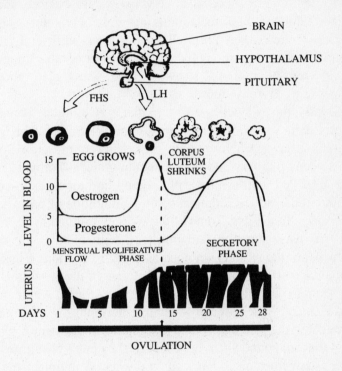

Figure 7: Normal menstrual cycle. (Reprinted with permission from Kate Neil, Balancing Hormones Naturally *[London: ION Press, 1994]).*

As might be imagined, the complete mechanism of the action of this vital nucleus within the hypothalamus is beyond present knowledge. It might help, however, to realize that the limbic brain, of which the hypothalamus is a part, is a biofeedback information and control center, with multiple neural centers sharing and integrating myriad biochemical, hormonal, immunologic, and emotional conditions. It functions as a giant analog computer complex with the capacity to formulate and send signals to the pituitary, as well as to control our autonomic nervous system balance and im-munomodulators, and create for us our sense of emotions and their physiologic responses. When all this is grasped sufficiently, it is no wonder that menstruation (and a great number of other things) can be affected by emotional states of mind, stress, diet, other hor-mones (e.g., thyroid), illness, or drugs of all sorts.

Clearly, this is a delicate system that is best not tampered with unless there's a good reason to do so. Yet this system is pro-foundly affected when synthetic progestins are prescribed. When the various pituitary and hypothalamic gonadal hormone recep-tors are filled with synthetically altered hormones, as in contra-ceptive pills and HRT, the net result is inhibition of one's natural hormones. In the past, some of these drugs resulted in permanent loss of ovary function (amenorrhea), with often tragic conse-quences for the women who had used them. The long lists of po-tential side effects for each and every one of the progestins does not seem to deter their use. The confusion wrought within the hy-pothalamus by the absence of the true hormones will reverberate throughout the province of this remarkable limbic center, with ef-fects that are bound *not* to be recognized by one's physician. Lim-bic system imbalance can lead to decreased immune response, decreased adrenal response, sleep disorders, peptic ulcers, de-pression, anxiety, panic, rage, learning disorders, and hormone disorders.

ANOVULATORY CYCLES

There is also the problem of anovulatory cycles, or cycles in which premenopausal women do not ovulate even though they continue to menstruate. This is known to occur in women athletes undergoing strenuous physical training, who may stop menstruating altogether. Anovulatory cycles also occur in nonexercising women, as is becoming evident through the many doctors such as myself who have tested progesterone levels in women. For example, Dr. Peter Ellison of Harvard University tested salivary hormone levels in eighteen regularly cycling, sexually active women, average age 29, and found that seven of them were not ovulating. I believe anovulatory cycles are epidemic among women in the industrialized countries. While factors such as nutrition, stress, and overexercising may be implicated, the most important factor for anovulatory cycles is most likely to be our xenoestrogen exposure. Without ovulation, no corpus luteum results and no progesterone is made. The graph below depicts hormone levels during anovulatory periods when no progesterone is produced:

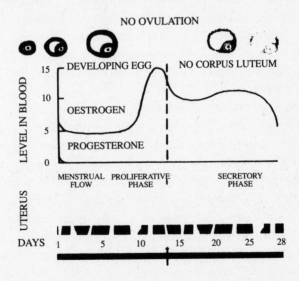

Figure 8: Hormone levels during an anovulatory menstrual cycle. (Reprinted with permission from Kate Neil, Balancing Hormones Naturally *[London: ION Press, 1994]).*

Several problems can result from anovulatory cycles. One is the monthlong presence of unopposed estrogen with all its attendant side effects, including the syndrome known as PMS. Another is the present, generally unrecognized problem of progesterone's role in osteoporosis. Contemporary medicine is still unaware that progesterone stimulates new bone formation. A third is the interrelationship between progesterone loss and stress. Stress influences limbic brain function, including the functioning of the hypothalamus. In brief, stress (and a bad diet) can also induce anovulatory cycles. The consequent lack of progesterone interferes with adrenal corticosteroid production by which one normally responds to stress. The effects of stress are therefore heightened, predisposing one to anovulatory cycles, creating the ultimate vicious cycle.

It should be obvious that hormone balance cannot be achieved if doctors continue to ignore the problem of progesterone deficiency. Since progesterone levels are rarely measured, most doctors are unaware that their menstruating patients may be deficient in progesterone. Adding estrogen and tranquilizers will not solve their problems.

An equally obvious corollary is that we must decrease our exposure to xenoestrogens. This requires several steps: (1) increased education on the dangers and sources of xenoestrogens; (2) decreased use of xenoestrogens such as petrochemical pesticides, PCB plastics, and some volatile solvents; and (3) learning to eat foods that not only have a lower load of petrochemical xenoestrogens but are good sources of phytoestrogens, the benign, weakly acting estrogenic compounds from plants that will compete at the receptor sites, thus protecting us from the more toxic petrochemical estrogenic compounds.

Given the complexity and heterogenicity (i.e., multiple factors) of cause and effect in the intricate arrangement of stress, diet, hypothalamic and pituitary function, and normal hormones, the prevailing attitude that female health concerns are merely a matter of estrogen "deficiency" is flawed, oversimplified, and ultimately dangerous. The progesterone factor can no longer be ignored. Women are right to be upset with their doctors for patting them on the head and sending them home with a prescription for synthetic hormones or tranquilizers.

PART II

Hormone Balance and Illness

Chapter 10

PROGESTERONE AND MENOPAUSE SYMPTOMS

This should have been the easiest chapter to write. After all, menopause symptoms are the defining characteristic of the menopause "problem." Yet much mystery prevails. Not all women passing through menopause have any of the usual panoply of symptoms, and the characteristic symptoms that some U.S. women and women in industrialized countries have are rare in third-world cultures. Though solid statistics are hard to validate, medical authorities teach that about 50 percent of women in the United States experience some degree of hot flashes during menopause, and only 15 percent seek medical treatment for them. Yet all women who go through menopause experience a drop in estrogen. Why do only some of them experience menopausal symptoms? Why do menopausal women in other cultures not experience these symptoms?

Early in my career, when I still felt assured of the medical education I had received and before I knew anything about natural progesterone, I was visited by a patient who first brought home to me the inadequacy of mainstream medical treatments. She was a sixty-two-year-old lady with persistent, quite severe hot flashes despite years of estrogen replacement therapy. She could tolerate the hot flashes but, as she apologetically explained, she was worried about the loss of libido, her inability to lose weight, and the thinning of her scalp hair. She was overweight and aware that the more estrogen she took the fatter she got and the more water she retained.

My medical examination and laboratory workup found nothing abnormal. In my naïveté, I thought I would be able to help her. I put her on my favorite low-fat, low sugar diet, added small doses of essential vitamin and mineral supplements, and tried manipulating her estrogen supplements to avoid water retention and fat buildup. Nothing I did helped her. With estrogen she had normal vaginal lubrication, but she still had hot flashes and her libido was just not there.

But failure is often a better instructor than success. So although I unfortunately wasn't much help to this patient, *she* was a help to *me*. In my attempt to unravel this knotty problem, I came to learn several important lessons: One, not all women with hot flashes are helped by supplemental estrogen. Two, fat increases estrogen levels in postmenopausal women. Three, fatter postmenopausal women generally have higher estrogen levels than thinner women. Four, postmenopausal women with normal estrogen levels can suffer hot flashes. Something more than estrogen deficiency is going on.

Let us look again at the symptoms associated with menopause for some women. Such a list would include:

- Hot flashes
- Vaginal dryness and atrophy
- Water retention

- Fat and weight gain, especially in the hips, thighs, and abdomen
- Sleep disturbances (insomnia, less REM-time sleep)
- Decreased libido
- Mood swings—depression, irritability
- Headaches, fatigue
- Short-term memory lapses, lack of concentration
- Dry, thin, wrinkly skin
- Thinning of scalp hair, some increase of facial hair
- Bone mineral loss (osteoporosis)
- Diffuse body aches and pains

THE MYSTERY OF MENOPAUSE

I know this will sound implausible, but the truth is that we don't really fully understand what happens during menopause and precisely why the menstrual cycle winds down. The prevailing medical view of menopause is that when a woman runs out of eggs, she stops menstruating and goes into menopause. Strangely enough, however, this is largely theory. The prevailing theory goes that a woman is born with all her follicles (from which eggs can be matured) already formed. Of the millions of follicles present before birth, about 300,000 are present at puberty. With every menstrual cycle, even those cycles when ovulation is suppressed by birth control hormones, hundreds of eggs vanish. When only about 1000 eggs are left, ovulation rarely occurs, even though estrogen production may remain adequate for menstruation. Thus such women continue menstruating and are in a state of estrogen dominance. In other words, loss of fertility is due to the disappearance of follicles and their eggs rather than age per se.

The cause or causes of actual menopause are still unclear. In some women, the hypothalamus stops producing GnRH—

presumably a genetically programmed change—whereas in many others, GnRH and the pituitary hormones, FSH and LH, continue being produced at regular levels and yet the ovaries do not or cannot respond. This latter situation is the one in which hot flashes are more likely to occur. The ovary is the weak link in the cycle of events. While poor nutrition and stress have traditionally been blamed, the more likely cause is xenoestrogen-caused ovarian dysfunction, a circumstance not anticipated by Mother Nature.

Fertility is also a function of the number of mature eggs a woman produces each month. Regardless of how many times a couple has sexual intercourse, the monthly probability of a 38-year-old woman conceiving is only about one-fourth that in a woman under age 30 because she is releasing fewer eggs or none at all.

The incidence of birth defects also rises as women and men age, although the exact mechanism of how this happens is not clearly understood.

A BRIEF LOOK AT PREMENOPAUSE

Menopausal symptoms may begin as much as a decade before menstruation stops altogether. This is due to the increasing numbers of women who are having anovulatory (nonovulating) cycles beginning in their midthirties. When this happens, they may menstruate but not ovulate. As we have seen, most progesterone is produced by the corpus luteum, itself formed at the time of ovulation. If there is no ovulation, progesterone levels drop dramatically. If there is too little progesterone, then estrogen dominates the hormonal environment. Anovulatory cycles may be regular or irregular, though often a woman notices that her menstrual flow is different, usually heavier or longer. (Premenopause syndrome will be covered in more detail in the following chapter.)

Low premenopausal progesterone caused by anovulatory cycles may lead to estrogen dominance prior to menopause. It is interesting to note that the most common age for the initial stages of breast or uterine cancer is five years or more *before* menopause, well before estrogen levels fall, but coinciding with a drop in progesterone.

(Note: If your physician wants to test you to find out whether you are ovulating, it can be revealed by testing for low serum or saliva progesterone levels during days 18 to 26 of the menstrual cycle.)

FALLING ESTROGEN AND PROGESTERONE, RISING GnRH, AND HOT FLASHES

Around age 45 to 50, sometimes a little earlier or later, estrogen levels begin to fall. When they fall below the levels necessary to signal the uterine lining to thicken and gather blood, the menstrual flow becomes less and/or irregular, eventually stopping altogether.

Let's zero in and take a closer look at hot flashes, the hallmark of menopausal symptoms. The prevailing explanation for hot flashes is as follows: Recall that an area (which we'll call the GnRH center) in the brain's hypothalamus monitors estrogen and progesterone levels. When levels fall, this center makes GnRH, which stimulates the pituitary to make hormones (FSH and LH), which in turn result in the ovarian production of estrogen and progesterone. The rise in these hormones inhibits further production of GnRH. At menopause, estrogen levels fall and progesterone levels are usually already low. The ovaries no longer respond to the FSH and LH prompt.

When a woman's ovaries *don't* respond to the FSH and LH signals by ovulating, the hormone signaling system can go awry. In effect, the hypothalamus begins "shouting," trying to tell the pituitary to tell the ovaries to ovulate. The inability of the ovaries to respond is most likely due to a final depletion of eggs and their surrounding follicle cells. This overactivity of the hypothalamus and pituitary signal begins affecting adjacent areas of the brain, which we'll call the vasomotor center (specifically the arcuate nucleus of the hypothalamus that controls capillary dilation and sweating mechanisms), and these are the women who get hot flashes. In addition to hot flashes, the heightened activity of the hypothalamus can cause mood swings, fatigue, feelings of being cold, and inappropriate responses to other stressors. Many women will have symptoms of hypothyroidism despite normal thyroid hormone levels.

In a nutshell:

1. The GnRH center effectively signals to increase estrogen and progesterone synthesis.
2. Elevated estrogen and progesterone inhibit GnRH release.
3. After menopause, the ovaries no longer make estrogen and progesterone.
4. Lack of estrogen and progesterone response results in increased activity of the GnRH center.
5. Heightened GnRH activity activates the vasomotor center, causing hot flashes and perspiration.

It is important to recognize that the GnRH center monitors both estrogen and progesterone. Thus, since the postmenopausal woman continues to make estrogen in respectable levels and makes little or no progesterone, hot flashes may well respond to progesterone supplementation alone. Hot flashes will also respond to much smaller doses of supplemental estrogen when progesterone is added. Even synthetic progestins like Provera (medroxyprogesterone acetate) or Megace (megestrol acetate) have been found effective in treating hot flashes, further indicating that estrogen per se is not the only factor in hot flashes.

The truth is that estrogen is only one part of the menopause picture and is certainly not a cure-all. In fact, these days I hear more complaints about the side effects of taking estrogen than I do about menopausal symptoms.

PROGESTERONE DEFICIENCY

If so much of a woman's health depends on a consistent level of progesterone, why does progesterone deficiency occur at menopause in Western societies? Did Mother Nature make a mistake? Mother Nature did not make the mistake; we did. Many plants (over 5000 known) make sterols that have progestogenic effects. In nonindustrialized cultures not subjected to xenoestrogens and whose diets are rich in fresh vegetables of all sorts, progesterone deficiency is rare. Not only do the majority of women in these cultures have healthy ovaries with healthy follicles producing sufficient progesterone, but at menopause their diets provide sufficient progestogenic substances to keep their sex drive high, their bones strong, and their passage through menopause uneventful and symptom-free.

Our food supply system uses many processed foods and foods that are picked days before being sold. Their vitamin (especially vitamin C) content and their sterol levels fall. We do not receive the progestogenic substances our forebears did. A *Lancet* article reported that the bone mineral density of skeletons from a church in England dating back to 1729 showed better bones at all ages compared to our skeletons of today. It is likely that both exercise and diet had something to do with that.

A drop in progesterone can cause a concurrent drop in corticosteroid production, leading to a whole other set of symptoms.

As you can see in Figure 9 on page 126, progesterone is a major precursor of the important corticosteroid hormones aldosterone and cortisol, made in the adrenal cortex. These corticosteroids are not made via any other hormone pathway. They are responsible for mineral balance, sugar control, and response to stresses of all sorts, including trauma, inflammation, and emotional stress. A lack of corticosteroids can lead to fatigue, immune dysfunction, hypoglycemia, allergies, and arthritis. Not infrequently, progesterone supplementation effectively resolves these problems.

The adrenal cortex is also capable of making progesterone, principally for its precursor role in making corticosteroids, but many women are so stressed out trying to work, raise children, and be wives that by the time they're in their mid- to late thirties or early forties their adrenal glands have nothing left to give. My guess is that when Western women stop making progesterone in their ovaries and their adrenal cortex and brain need to pick up 100 percent of that function to produce corticosteroids, there isn't much progesterone left over for other functions, such as balancing estrogen levels. The adrenals of many women in Western cultures are so depleted they can't even make enough progesterone to make the corticosteroids. This may be an important factor in chronic fatigue syndrome, which is so common in women in their midthirties and early forties.

MENOPAUSE AND ESTROGEN

Remember, the prevailing myth in mainstream medicine is that menopause is an estrogen deficiency disease, but estrogen levels drop only 40 to 60 percent at menopause, while progesterone levels can drop to nearly zero.

One of the paradoxes of the delicate dance of hormones in a woman's body is that estrogen and progesterone, though mutually antagonistic in some of their effects, each sensitize receptor sites for the other. That is, the presence of estrogen makes body target tissues more sensitive to progesterone, and the presence of progesterone does the same for estrogen. Each sets the stage for the body to be more responsive to the other—an interesting example of nature's efficiency.

Progesterone has an opposing, or balancing, effect on estrogen. When progesterone levels drop to near zero, we have estrogen dominance, which causes a long list of unpleasant symptoms. Estrogen dominance does not necessarily mean a woman has too much estrogen; it simply means that estrogen levels are *relatively* higher than progesterone, creating a hormonal imbalance with its attendant estrogenic side effects.

Estrogen proponents, such as Judith Reichman, M.D., an active popularizer of ERT, argue that hot flashes during the night interrupt sleep and this leads to the mood swings, fatigue, and memory and concentration problems. With ERT all problems are eliminated, she claims. In my thirty years of practice, I found this is not the case. Sleep interruption may well play a part in these symptoms, but the many women I saw in practice with persistent symptoms despite estrogen replacement tell me that estrogen is not the cure-all as claimed. Something more is going on. When I added transdermal natural progesterone in physiologic dosages to their medical treatment, remarkable improvement invariably occurred.

Unopposed estrogen (i.e., lacking progesterone) carries health risks itself. Mainstream medicine acknowledges that unopposed estrogen greatly increases the risk of endometrial cancer, for instance, and probably promotes breast cancer. Not yet generally understood is that estrogen alters cell membrane function such that sodium and water influxes into body cells, while potassium and magnesium are lost from cells. This results in intracellular edema or bloating and water retention. Estrogen also promotes abnormal cellular retention of copper and loss of zinc. These important changes in intracellular electrolytes and cellular edema go a long way to explain mood swings, loss of concentration, and the aches and pains that menopausal women suffer from, even with estrogen replacement. Progesterone, on the other hand, works to protect the cell membrane from these estrogen-induced problems.

ANDROGENS AND MENOPAUSE

Androgens are hormones that have masculinizing effects. In women they are made primarily in the ovaries and adrenal glands. Androgen hormones include testosterone, dihydrotestosterone, androstanediol, androstenediol, and two weakly androgenic hormones, androstenedione and dehydroepiandrosterone (DHEA). The precursor hormone to the androgens is pregnenolone, which then follows a pathway either through progesterone or DHEA. We'll call these the "progesterone" pathway or the "DHEA" pathway.

A simplified diagram of the two pathways follows:

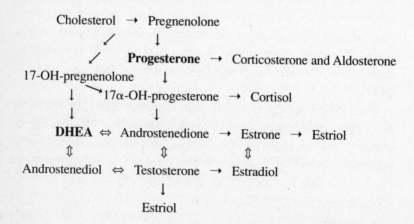

Figure 9: The progesterone and DHEA hormone synthesis pathways.

The DHEA pathway is more active in males than females and can occur in both the testes and adrenals. In ovulating women, both pathways are operative. However, in the ovaries a highly active enzyme called aromatase rapidly converts androgens into estrogen, thus sparing women the masculinizing effects of the androgens. At menopause, when ovary function slows, the adrenal DHEA pathway becomes more active in women. They may experience symptoms of hair loss on the head and the growth of coarser hair on the face and arms (hirsutism), caused by a shift in hormone pathways that favors the androgens. Their body fat becomes a reservoir for the major androgens, some of which are converted into estrone, an estrogen. In women with ample body fat, significant amounts of estrone can be obtained by conversion from fat-stored androgens. Be that as it may, the fact is that after menopause, androgen/estrogen ratios shift in favor of androgens, often leading to increased facial and body hair and male pattern baldness. My clinical experience is that progesterone supplementation often results in the disappearance of facial hair and the regrowth of scalp hair. Why should this be?

The most active of the androgens is testosterone, which also is a product of the adrenal DHEA pathway. In women, about 99 percent of their testosterone is bound to other substances and thus is unavailable as an active hormone. The rate at which available testosterone is cleared from a woman's body is related to her hormone balance. Estrogen decreases testosterone clearance whereas progesterone increases it. Thus, when estrogen is dominant, testosterone clearance is decreased, increasing the effect of available testosterone. When progesterone is added, the clearance of testosterone is increased and its androgenic effects are reduced.

WHAT CAN BE DONE FOR MENOPAUSAL SYMPTOMS?

The common thread running through all these conditions is estrogen dominance in relationship to a relative insufficiency of progesterone. At this point, the last thing a woman needs is more estrogen!

The vast majority of menopausal problems can be avoided by good nutrition, avoidance of toxins, regular exercise, and the proper supplementation, when indicated for hormone balance, of real, honest-to-God, natural progesterone. A very small percentage of women continue to have hot flashes and vaginal dryness. Once again, I have found that a few months or at most a year or two on natural estrone or estriol solves that problem. Estriol is the predominant estrogen made by the placenta when the ovaries are resting during pregnancy. I will describe a natural hormone balance program and how to use natural progesterone in Chapters 18 and 19.

Chapter 11

HORMONE BALANCE, PREMENOPAUSE SYNDROME, AND THE ADRENAL AND THYROID GLANDS

When it takes place as nature intended, menopause isn't a sudden stopping of menstrual periods. It isn't an event, like a birthday. It's a long, gradual process of lowering hormone levels. Eventually hormone levels drop below the point necessary to create a menstrual cycle. Throughout the book so far I've been alluding to the period of time in a woman's life called premenopause (perimenopause to doctors), the decade or so before menopause when a woman's reproductive functions are winding down. In agrarian, nonindustrialized cultures, this is an uneventful time. In Western, industrialized countries, it's a time when increasing numbers of women suffer from chronic fatigue, weight gain, mood swings, unstable blood sugar, and rapid aging. Women who have waited to have children may find they are infertile. I call this premenopause syndrome. What has gone awry?

PREMENOPAUSE SYNDROME

There are clear physiological and biochemical reasons for premenopause syndrome, but the whole woman—including the emotional, mental, and spiritual aspects—needs to be taken into account if we are to get to the root causes. At the risk of sounding unscientific, let's first look at the female body in a way that owes much to Chinese medicine and the concepts of yin and yang. This will be a simplified explanation, but it will suffice for the purposes of illustrating my point.

In its essence the female body is yin and the male body is yang. Each contains some of the other, but yin predominates for females and yang predominates for males. Yin is dark and earthy. The yin personality would tend to be nurturing, passive, introverted, calm, intuitive, and soft.

Yang is light and abstract. The yang personality would tend to be active, outgoing, focused, aggressive, logical, and impatient.

Estrogens, the hormones responsible for female sexual development, and progesterone, the progestational, or mothering, hormone, tend to produce yin behavior. Testosterone and DHEA, two of the hormones responsible for male sexual development, tend to produce yang behavior. Although generalizations are always untrue by their very nature, women tend to "default" more on the side of yin behavior and men tend to "default" more on the side of yang behavior.

The environment of raising children naturally favors the yin or female attributes. The business world naturally favors the yang or male attributes. What happens when a woman finds herself spending her days in an environment that's very yang, as so many working women do these days? To survive and thrive, she is going to minimize her yin aspects and maximize her yang aspects. Her body will pay attention to these signals and respond accordingly. The stereotype successful woman executive is slim, trim, and muscular—yang. The stereotype mother figure is ample in breasts, hips, and thighs—yin. These differences in roles work fine when a woman's life is balanced, when she has ample time and energy to develop both sides. But take a woman who is working full-time, has a couple of kids, and a husband who also works and we have a recipe for imbalance and stress. This woman is going to be pulling on her yang attributes at the expense of her yin attributes. She's likely to be chronically exhausted, always "on," never taking time for herself. She is constantly forced to push the limits of her endurance to keep up. She rarely has time to spend quiet, nurturing time with her children or herself, not to mention her husband. In an effort just to maintain her lifestyle, her adrenal glands are constantly pumping out hormones meant to be used sparingly for "fight or flight" situations and they eventually become tired, sluggish, and depleted. Her body gets the message that survival is at stake. Blood sugar becomes constantly unstable. Digestion goes awry so she isn't absorbing nutrients properly. The ovaries respond by shutting down in favor of survival. When her ovaries shut down, progesterone production occurs only at the adrenals, but they aren't working and she's not getting any progesterone from poor dietary habits, so she becomes progesterone-deficient and estrogen dominant.

The estrogen dominance causes the all-too-familiar signs of fatigue, depression, little or no desire for sex, weight gain, water retention, headaches, and mood swings. By her late thirties and early forties, she probably has fibrocystic breasts, uterine fibroids, or endometriosis. The estrogen dominance interferes with thyroid action, which increases her fatigue, so she's cold all the time and she's gaining more weight. But her doctor gives her a thyroid function test and it comes out normal; she produces the normal amount of thyroid, but it's not being used effectively. Not realizing the role of estrogen dominance, her doctor often prescribes thyroid supplements.

She diets continuously (bingeing in between on sugar, caffeine, and refined carbohydrates in a desperate attempt to get her adrenals jump-started), but it does no good because her metabolism has also gone into survival mode, which is to say it's very, very slow. Due to her sluggish adrenals, she finds it very difficult to get out of bed in the morning. Does this sound familiar? It's an all-too-common scenario. In fact I would venture to say it's epidemic among working mothers in their thirties and forties. But premenopause syndrome is by no means limited to working mothers. Even without children, women who get on a career track and develop their yang attributes at the expense of their yin attributes are likely to suffer from hormone imbalances.

Another major source of hormonal stress is the xenoestrogens. As I mentioned earlier, people living in an industrialized culture are continuously exposed to environmental sources of petrochemical derivatives that convey potent "estrogenic" actions. These sources include pesticides, herbicides, auto pollution, polycyclic aromatic hydrocarbons (PAHs), polychlorinated biphenyls (PCBs), and nonylphenols (alkylphenol polyethoxylates or APEs) found in many detergents. In females, the results may be enlarged ovaries, possible ovarian tumors, breast cancer, and premature "burnout" of ovarian follicles, contributing to premenopause syndrome. In males, the results include atrophy of testes, reduced sperm counts, small penises, and possibly prostate cancer.

To add insult to injury, once anovulatory cycles begin, the insidious process of osteoporosis follows. Progesterone, the bone-building hormone, is missing. Poor diet and lack of exercise are pulling calcium off the bone faster than it can be put on. Many women arrive at menopause with osteoporosis well under way, already having lost 25 to 30 percent of their bone mass.

FOLLICLE BURNOUT

The two primary causes of premenopause syndrome are anovulatory cycles and adrenal exhaustion. It's hard to say which comes first. Anovulatory cycles are those in which a woman does not ovulate. No egg is released into the fallopian tube for its journey to the uterus and no progesterone is produced. The anovulatory woman will still menstruate because the estrogen is still present, but her progesterone levels will be low because there is no corpus luteum present to produce it. Anovulatory cycles are becoming common in women in their midthirties long before actual menopause. Dr. Jerilynn Prior, professor of endocrinology at the University of British Columbia in Vancouver, British Columbia, Canada, found that it was very common for women athletes (who developed osteoporosis despite normal estrogen levels) to have anovulatory periods. If they were training hard enough, eventually even their periods would stop. However, when Prior went out to find a control group of "normal" women for her studies, she discovered that anovulatory cycles among women from their midthirties through forties was quite common. When Drs. Ben C. Campbell and Peter T. Ellison tested menstrual variation in salivary testosterone among regularly cycling women ages 24 to 42 (average age 29), they also tested salivary progesterone during the luteal phase and found seven of the 18 subjects were not ovulating. More and more women are truly progesterone-deficient prior to menopause.

The constellation of stress, poor diet, exposure to xenoestrogens, and progesterone deficiency is very likely the cause of what we call the premenopause syndrome. Furthermore, the xenoestrogens very likely contribute to endometrial, ovarian, and breast cancer.

ESTROGEN EXCESS

Not only is progesterone deficiency common during the premenopause years, but estrogen levels tend to fluctuate and become excessive. Two causes for this are higher FSH levels and a
matter of energetics. When women with symptoms of premenopause syndrome arrive at a physician's office, frequently a
lab test for estradiol, FSH, and LH is ordered. Because progesterone is low, FSH levels may be high. The increased FSH levels
result in increased ovarian production of estrogen but not of progesterone, because of follicle depletion. The attempt of the hypothalamus to restore hormone balance is subverted by the follicle
depletion and leads instead to increased estrogen dominance.
Most physicians, however, are unaware of the follicle depletion
and interpret the test to mean merely that the patient is not yet
truly menopausal.

Other researchers such as Dr. Ellison point out another possible
mechanism for this estrogen excess that characterizes premenopausal women in industrialized countries. It has been found
that when energy intake is low (insufficient dietary calories) and
energy requirements are high (more physical labor), women's estrogen levels fall, often to such low levels that fertility is impaired.
That is, during starvation periods, birth rates fall. Conversely,
when energy intake is high and energy requirements are low, estrogen levels rise, often to levels considerably higher than that
found in third-world cultures. This excess estrogen frequently
produces heavy irregular menstrual bleeding as well as a host of
other symptoms reflecting unopposed estrogen side effects.

In my practice over the years, serum estrogen levels taken during these premenopause years reveal great variability, not only
from person to person but also in any given woman when such
tests are taken randomly.

A premenopausal woman from New York called me to ask

what her recently taken estrogen level might mean. When I told her of the day-to-day and week-to-week variability of estrogen levels during the premenopausal years, she talked her doctor into ordering a series of weekly estrogen levels during the weeks between her periods. She called back later to report that her serum estrogen levels varied from a low of 11 to a high of 300 picograms/milliliter, with levels of 60 and 220 in between, none of them appropriate for the time of her menstrual month. She also reported that her doctor was mystified, saying he'd never seen anything like this before. I asked if her doctor had ever done serial tests on anyone before!

Thus, among premenopausal women in industrialized countries, there exist variable inappropriate surges of estrogen, a generally higher-than-normal level of estrogen, and a generally unrecognized epidemic of progesterone deficiency. Each of these contributes to the remarkable incidence of premenopausal symptoms we see in the United States and other industrialized countries.

SYMPTOMS OF PREMENOPAUSE SYNDROME

Fatigue
Depression
Weight gain
Water retention
Headaches
Loss of sex drive
Mood swings
Inability to handle stress
Irritability
Fibrocystic breasts
Uterine fibroids

Endometriosis
Low metabolism
Symptoms of hypothyroidism with normal T3 and T4 levels
Unstable blood sugar
Craving for caffeine, sweets, and carbohydrates
Sluggishness in the morning

THE ADRENAL GLANDS

The adrenals are two small glands about the size and shape of a flattened prune that sit on top of the kidneys. Each adrenal gland is composed of an outer and inner part: the outer cortex and the inner medulla. Both the medulla and the cortex produce important secretions that are part of our stress reactions.

The adrenal medulla plays a role in regulating the sympathetic nervous system: It speeds up the heart rate, narrows blood vessels, and raises blood pressure and blood sugar by secreting two hormones called epinephrine (also called adrenaline) and norepinephrine (noradrenaline). You probably recognize the name epinephrine because synthetic variations of this hormone are found in over-the-counter cold and allergy remedies that work by narrowing blood vessels. Epinephrine is the hormone secreted when you're under stress, inducing Hans Selye's now famous "fight or flight" reaction in the body that our ancestors evolved to help them survive by fleeing or fighting off attackers. When epinephrine is released, many things occur simultaneously and quickly in the body: The heart speeds up; blood is sent flooding into the heart, lungs, muscles, and brain and away from the digestive system; sugar is dumped into the blood in large quantities to provide quick energy; and breathing is faster. This is a great system if you need to run from or turn and fight a saber-toothed tiger. If your boss is yelling at you, the fight or flight response still occurs, but its manifestations are suppressed by "higher" parts of your brain telling you that fleeing or physically fighting are counterproductive in that situation. Your body is flooded with contradictory messages and reactions. This in itself is a factor in disease, eventual fatigue, and physical illness.

Events that provoke a fight or flight response are called stressors. Stress is a household word these days—we all have it to one degree or another. We have the day-to-day stressors of hectic schedules, traffic jams, colds and flus, pressure on the job, mechanical breakdowns, and troublesome relationships. Then we have the big stressors such as the death or serious illness of a loved one, losing or gaining a job, moving, having a child, marriage, divorce, and so forth. Any of these types of stressors can send the adrenal medulla into action with epinephrine.

To go back to the yin and yang metaphor, epinephrine is a very yang hormone. When we're stimulated by it we tend to be very alert, focused, and energetic. This type of energy is particularly valued in the business world. Some people will work themselves into an anger or fear response just to get a "hit" of epinephrine. The bad news is that epinephrine is not a hormone meant to be used all the time—it's designed to be used in emergencies for short bursts of intense energy. If we're always calling on our epinephrine to get us up and going, eventually we fall prey to an imbalance and our adrenal medulla becomes exhausted.

THE ADRENAL CORTEX

The adrenal cortex secretes three classes of hormones—glucocorticoids, mineralcorticoids, and androgens—that play literally dozens of ongoing roles in regulating bodily functions. While the secretions of the adrenal medulla provide quick and short-term responses to immediate stress, the adrenal cortex hormones provide longer-term responses for stress and homeostasis, the maintenance of balance in bodily functions. The adrenal cortex hormones are often considered essential for life. Animals with their adrenal glands removed will survive for a long time if maintained in an environment providing proper nutrition and freedom from stress. However, if put to any significant stress such as infection, trauma, hunger, or fatigue, they will quickly die. Adrenal cortical hormones are essential for life because life as we know it is stressful. Let us take a closer look at the three adrenal cortex hormones.

The most important glucocorticoids are cortisol and hydrocortisone, which play a role in regulating blood sugar, how carbohydrates, proteins, and fats are moved in and out of cells, inflammation, and muscle function. If too many cortisols are present (as from adrenal cortical tumors or pharmaceutical dosages of cortisol medication), the symptoms are weight gain (especially around the midsection), blood sugar imbalances, thinning skin, muscle wasting, and other signs of aging. Women whose glucocorticoid pathways are not functioning properly or who are deficient in the cortisols (as from adrenal exhaustion or lack of adrenal reserve after overly prolonged stress or malnutrition) may have fatigue, low blood sugar, and sometimes weight loss and menstrual dysfunction.

The mineralcorticoids, especially aldosterone, regulate the balance of minerals in the cells, mainly sodium and potassium, but magnesium is also affected. Stress triggers the release of aldosterone, which raises blood pressure by its action on body cells to hold onto sodium and lose potassium and magnesium. Long-term release of stress-level mineralcorticoids can cause a potassium deficiency and a magnesium imbalance as well as chronic water retention and high blood pressure. Magnesium loss is an exceedingly important factor in our overall health, being the most common cofactor for optimal enzyme function, but magnesium deficiency is not commonly recognized by standard blood tests. Since it is predominantly an intracellular mineral, standard serum (the watery, noncellular part of blood) tests do not adequately measure magnesium. A red blood cell magnesium level test is better.

The adrenal cortex also makes all of the sex hormones, but in very small amounts. One cortical hormone, DHEA, which is weakly androgenic, is made in large amounts in both men and women; its production is greater than that of any of the other corticosteroids. Its full range of functions is yet to be understood. It will be discussed more completely below. The sex hormones, as you have discovered in reading about estrogen and progesterone, play a part in regulating many bodily functions and are inextricably bound up with the balance of the adrenal hormones.

As you can see from Figure 9 on page 126, cholesterol is a precursor to all of the adrenal cortex and sex hormones, and progesterone is a precursor to aldosterone, the mineralcorticoid that regulates fluids in your cells, and cortisol. This means that aldosterone and cortisol are made from progesterone. Now that you know how important aldosterone and cortisol are to bodily functions, you can imagine what havoc a deficiency of progesterone can wreak on hormone balance and bodily functions. It's no wonder that progesterone-deficient women are suffering from so many illnesses.

You can also now understand how chronic stress can cause hormone imbalances and may even contribute to a deficiency of progesterone, as it is used for "survival," meaning the production of adrenal hormones, rather than contributing to all the hormone pathways, in particular balancing and opposing estrogen.

THE ROLE OF DHEA

DHEA (dehydroepiandrosterone) and DHEA-S (a sulfated counterpart) are the most abundantly produced steroid hormones in the body. (See the appendix on page 356 for a molecular diagram of DHEA and DHEA-S.) DHEA is important to the growth and repair of protein tissues. The full spectrum of its actions is not yet completely known. It is especially important during pregnancy, when the placenta becomes the major source of both estrogen and progesterone. However, the placenta cannot make estrogen in the same way the ovary does during menstrual cycles. Instead of making it from progesterone, the placenta makes estrogen from the mother's adrenal DHEA-S. As the pregnancy proceeds, more DHEA-S is also made by the fetus's adrenals. In addition, the fetus's liver changes the DHEA-S to 16α-OH-DHEA, which is used by the placenta as the precursor for estriol, which in turn becomes the major estrogen produced during pregnancy.

Blood levels of DHEA in men and women peak at around age 20 and then gradually decline with age. This decline in DHEA has been correlated by DHEA promoters with an increased risk of many degenerative diseases, including heart disease, breast cancer, diabetes, obesity, high blood pressure, and Parkinson's disease. However, it is not clear at this time whether DHEA plays a true preventative role in this correlation or whether it is merely a marker of increased risk.

Supplementation with DHEA is something of an alternative health fad right now, but it would behoove doctors to be cautious in its use with women. Some promoters claim that DHEA "burns" fat and therefore prevents and/or treats obesity. Most of the studies done have been on men, and many in the health care fields are making the mistake of thinking that what applies to a man applies to a woman. When it comes to how sex hormones behave, this is almost never true and DHEA is no exception. In premenopausal women, for example, high DHEA-S levels are associated with increased fat around the midsection and decreased leg fat accumulation, whereas no such effect is seen in men. In healthy *post*menopausal women, higher androgen levels (which are created by DHEA supplementation) are also associated with weight gain around the midsection and insulin resistance, whereas in men, higher androgen levels tend to correlate with less weight gain around the midsection. Because of their insulin resistance effect, both glucocorticoids and DHEA are contraindicated in people with diabetes, especially women.

There is also a mistaken notion that DHEA is a precursor to all of the adrenal and ovarian hormones when in fact it is primarily a precursor to androstenediol, testosterone, and the estrogens. It is *not* a precursor to pregnenolone, progesterone, the cortisols, or aldosterone. (See Figure 9.) And, in practice, DHEA rarely seems to act as an estrogen precursor in women; instead it goes down the androgen or male hormone pathways. Estrogen can be produced by conversion from androstenedione but the conversion rate is only about 1 percent.

The role of DHEA in breast cancer is also unclear. The risk of breast cancer is increased by androgen deficiency and estradiol (estrogen) excess. Increased risk of breast cancer is associated with low DHEA concentrations in premenopausal women and with high DHEA concentrations in postmenopausal women. In normal female rats, DHEA appears to inhibit the growth of breast cancer (mammary carcinoma), but in rats whose ovaries have been removed and who are estrogen deficient, DHEA stimulates tumor cell growth. It is clear that much research still needs to be done.

If progesterone is deficient in pre- and postmenopausal women, the DHEA pathway tends to take up the slack. However, most of it is not converted to estrogen and at higher doses, DHEA-induced androgens can lead to male pattern baldness, excessive facial hair growth, abdominal obesity, and, some studies suggest, an increased risk of heart disease and insulin resistance. My elderly women patients suffering from (probable) DHEA pathway dominance began to grow their scalp hair back and lose their facial hair with the regular use of natural progesterone.

Current research suggests that in men, DHEA, which is a direct precursor to testosterone, may be of value in preventing and treating cardiovascular disease, high cholesterol, diabetes, obesity, cancer, Alzheimer's disease, other memory disturbances, immune system disorders, chronic fatigue, and aging. In general I wouldn't recommend it for pre- or postmenopausal women, but it's possible that it could be effectively supplemented in small doses when needed without the undesirable side effects. As research progresses, I predict that DHEA will join progesterone, estrogen, and testosterone as an important hormone in its own right.

DHEA circulates in the blood primarily as DHEA-S, the sulfated version, which is not in itself biologically active—an important fact if your doctor is testing your DHEA levels. Blood plasma levels of DHEA-S can be considered a circulating reservoir from which the active form can be derived. Conversely, DHEA can be converted back to DHEA-S. Regulators of this conversion process are not known. When blood tests for DHEA are done, the test results do not usually discriminate between the 95 percent that is DHEA-S and the 5 percent that is DHEA. Radioimmune assays of saliva, however, can be used to measure the concentration of the biologically active hormone DHEA. (See page 334 for information on ordering saliva testing of hormone levels.)

Some consider the true "mother" sterol to be pregnenolone, which in the ovaries and adrenals is the precursor to both progesterone and DHEA. Since pregnenolone synthesis from cholesterol occurs in the mitochondria of all cells in the body and is not unique to the ovaries, testes, or adrenals, pregnenolone deficiency seems unlikely to me. Future research may reveal a role for pregnenolone not apparent at this time.

NUTRITIONAL ADRENAL SUPPORT

Not surprisingly, nutrition is as important to the adrenal glands as it is to all tissues of the body. But in the case of adrenal glands, vitamin C is uniquely important: Cells of adrenal glands use vitamin C at a higher rate than any other cells. Their use of vitamin C varies with their need, and their need rises when the body is required to respond to stress of any sort. It follows that vitamin C deficiency adversely impacts on adrenal gland performance. Chronic stress will more likely lead to adrenal exhaustion or lack of reserve ("lazy" adrenal gland function) if vitamin C levels are lower than optimal. The RDA (recommended daily allowance) of 60 milligrams per day for vitamin C intake is predicated on vitamin C need in healthy young adults without metabolic stress; this RDA is *not* appropriate for people under such stress as illness, infection, surgery, trauma, fatigue, or any metabolic or even psychological stress.

The vast majority of animals make their own vitamin C as needed. When put under stress, their vitamin C production increases. Humans are one of the few animals (along with Rhesus monkeys, guinea pigs, rind-eating bats of India, and parakeets) who do not make their own vitamin C and must therefore obtain it from diet or supplements. The typical animal with a metabolic rate similar to humans makes about four grams (one-eighth of an ounce or 4000 milligrams) daily per 100 pounds of body weight. During stress, their production can rise to 12 grams daily per 100 pounds of body weight. Since humans are part of the animal kingdom, it is likely that our vitamin C intake should approximate at least four grams per day to avoid stress-induced exhaustion of our adrenal glands. Even without undue stress, one's vitamin C intake should be one to two grams a day to maintain optimal levels. This is not easy to do through diet alone. An orange provides 60 milligrams of vitamin C. To achieve an intake of one gram (1000 milligrams) of vitamin C, one would have to eat approximately 18 oranges; thus the need for vitamin C supplements.

Metabolic stress from oxidation reactions is unavoidable. Numerous studies show the benefits of natural antioxidants. Our diet selections should include optimal antioxidants such as are found in unprocessed fruit and vegetables of all sorts. In addition, I routinely take 400 IU of vitamin E, 15 milligrams of beta carotene, and 60 micrograms of selenium. Bioflavonoids such as quercetin, which enhance vitamin C, can also be supplemented and are very effective for treating allergies.

A middle-aged woman came to me with a problem of advanced osteoporosis caused by ten years or so of cortisone medication taken for chronic asthma. She had shrunk about eight inches in height. Every attempt to wean her off cortisone had resulted in symptoms of Addison's disease—severe weakness as a result of adrenal gland failure—and a return of her asthma. Her adrenal cortex was so suppressed by the long-term use of cortisone medication that it could not return to function on its own, so to speak. She had been told that the cause of her allergic asthma was aspirin (acetyl-salicylate), which she strictly avoided. Nobody had told her of the salicylates found naturally in food. I provided her with a list of salicylate-containing foods to avoid and recommended vitamin C in divided doses to four grams total a day, plus progesterone cream for its important role as a precursor in cortisone synthesis. Then I instructed her to slowly reduce her cortisone medication dosage. Two months later she returned feeling well and off medication for the first time in ten years. With continued use of progesterone, her cortisone-induced bone loss abated and eventually her bones became stronger again, greatly reducing her risk of fracture.

Several lessons can be learned by examples such as this. Treating the disease's cause is better than treating its symptoms. The knowledge and application of nutrition is important to the health of all cells. Aiding normal health-giving mechanisms is better than suppressing normal functions. Our natural ability to heal and be well is far too great an asset to ignore (or inhibit).

PROGESTERONE AND THYROID HORMONE

Though each hormone is unique, hormone balance involves a complex harmonious blend of all hormones. I tend to think of hormones as instruments in an orchestra—the harmony we seek is the proper contribution of all the instruments together not only in pitch but also in volume and rhythm. The same is true of sex hormones and thyroid hormone.

In my medical practice, I was impressed with the much greater number of women taking thyroid supplements for hypothyroidism (low thyroid) than men. Thyroid is the hormone that regulates metabolic rate. Low thyroid tends to cause low energy levels, cold intolerance, and weight gain. Excess thyroid causes higher energy levels, feeling too warm, and weight loss.

The thyroid gland makes from tyrosine, one of the amino acids, and iodine, two versions of thyroid hormone, one containing four atoms of iodine (thyroxine, T4) and another version containing three atoms of iodine (triiodothyronine, T3). Both versions are then enveloped in a relatively large glycoprotein complex called thyroglobulin and stored in the thyroid gland.

To be released into the bloodstream for circulation throughout the body, the hormones are separated from thyroglobulin and bound to a much smaller globulin (thyroxine-binding globulin) or albumin. However, only 0.5 percent of thyroid hormone is "free" to be biologically active. It is the "free" hormone that can leave the bloodstream and enter body cells, where it meets with a special receptor and thereby modulates the cell's metabolic rate. Thyroid's action in the cell is to increase the biosynthesis of enzymes, resulting in heat production, oxygen consumption, and elevated metabolic rate. Thyroid stimulates the release of free fatty acids from adipose (fat) tissue, stimulates the oxidation of fatty acids (energy production), and reduces cholesterol by oxidizing it into bile acids. Thyroid also stimulates enzymes for protein synthesis and, when present in excessive amounts, can catabolize (destroy) muscle protein.

As with the sex hormones, a neural center in the hypothalamus monitors the blood level of T3 and T4. If the levels are low, the hypothalamus sends a message, thyrotropin-releasing hormone (TRH), to the pituitary, which then sends its message, thyrotropin, also known as thyroid-stimulating hormone (TSH), through the bloodstream to the thyroid gland to stimulate it to make more thyroid hormone. If the thyroid levels rise too high, the hypothalamus detects this and reduces or stops its TRH, which results in lower TSH and the consequent diminished production of thyroid hormone. This is the same negative feedback system our body uses to regulate sex hormone levels. What difference should gender make to the incidence of hypothyroidism?

As I became aware of estrogen dominance syndrome, I noticed that the taking of thyroid supplements was especially common in women with this condition. When I attempted to correct their estrogen dominance by adding progesterone, it was common to see that their need for thyroid supplements decreased and could often be successfully eliminated. Thus I became aware that estrogen, progesterone, and thyroid hormones are interrelated.

Many of these women had come to me from other doctors' offices for PMS or osteoporosis prevention and/or treatment. On reviewing the laboratory studies that had led to their presumed diagnosis of hypothyroidism, I often found that their T3 and T4 levels had been normal and their TSH levels only slightly elevated. Their thyroid supplement had been prescribed on the basis of hypothyroid-like symptoms such as feeling tired or sluggish, a little cold intolerance, and thinning hair, for example. While the thyroid medication had improved their tiredness a bit, it had not corrected the symptoms I had learned to associate with estrogen dominance such as fat and water retention, breast swelling, headaches, and loss of libido. When their hormones were balanced, meaning progesterone deficiency was adequately treated, not only did their estrogen dominance symptoms decrease or disappear but so did their presumed hypothyroidism!

Let us look at this situation again. Estrogen causes food calories to be stored as fat. Thyroid hormone causes fat calories to be turned into usable energy. Thyroid hormone and estrogen have opposing actions. The "central command post" of this opposition may be in the hypothalamus, the pituitary, the thyroid gland, or the body cells where the hormones enact their destined roles. My hypothesis is that estrogen inhibits thyroid action in the cells, probably interfering with the binding of thyroid to its receptor. Both hormones have phenol rings at a corner of their molecule. Estrogen may compete with thyroid hormone at the site of its receptor. In so doing, the thyroid hormone may never complete its mission, creating the hypothyroid symptoms despite normal serum levels of thyroid hormone. Progesterone, on the other hand, increases the sensitivity of estrogen receptors for estrogen and yet, at the proper level, inhibits many of estrogen's side effects. That is what is meant when we say that progesterone *opposes* estrogen: The lack of progesterone in a woman still making estrogen or taking estrogen supplements leads to the condition of *unopposed* estrogen.

I will leave the exact mechanism of action to the biochemists, but it is clear to me that symptoms of hypothyroidism occurring in patients with unopposed estrogen (progesterone-deficient) become less so when progesterone is added and hormone balance is attained.

Another common thyroid dysfunction is Hashimoto's thyroiditis, which is an autoimmune inflammatory process of the thyroid gland. That means the body is creating antibodies against the cells that make up the thyroid gland. The exact cause of this disease is unknown. However, inhibitory antibodies bind to TSH receptors, displacing TSH, and this may be at least one of the mechanisms by which this disorder results in inefficient production of thyroid hormone. As the disease progresses, cells of the thyroid gland are destroyed and inflammation occurs, along with fibrous deterioration of the entire gland.

Autoimmune disorders in general are thought to be triggered by transient viruses in susceptible people; the virus triggers antibodies against some protein component of the virus. By some probably minor fluke, the antibodies attack similar proteins in certain body tissues, in this case the thyroid. Corticosteroids block this attack by one's own antibodies. Diagnosis is made by detecting the presence and serum levels of the particular antibody. In some people, Hashimoto's thyroiditis also causes leakage of excess T3 and T4 into the serum, resulting in a hyperthyroid state (thyroidtoxicosis) usually of short duration. The usual treatment of Hashimoto's thyroiditis is suppression of gland function by full doses of thyroid medication, such as thyroxine and/or triiodothyronine.

It has been my experience in practice that when a woman with Hashimoto's thyroiditis is given progesterone for osteoporosis, for example, there results a gradual diminution in the severity and sometimes a complete resolution of the thyroiditis problem. One can hypothesize that estrogen dominance may have had a hand in triggering the errant antibodies and thus correcting the estrogen dominance leads to gradual correction of the problem.

Progesterone is also the main precursor of corticosteroids and in progesterone-deficient women, restoration of normal progesterone levels may enhance normal corticosteroid production, thus suppressing the autoimmune attack.

SUPPORTING YOUR THYROID GLAND WITH NUTRITION

The thyroid gland is a resilient gland; many people with terrible nutrition have normal functioning thyroid glands. However, several nutrients are important to proper thyroid gland function, and iodine, of course, is crucial. The synthesis and secretion of thyroid hormone requires sufficient amino acids (proteins) for normal albumin levels and, in particular, for tyrosine or the amino acids from which we can make tyrosine. The crucial nutrient for thyroid hormone synthesis is iodine. Before this was discovered, people living well away from the sea were prone to develop enlarged thyroid glands (goiter) and, in more advanced cases, cretinism (arrested physical and mental development with lowered metabolic rate) or myxedema (dry, waxy swelling of the skin and mucus membranes). Eventually it became clear that eating fish or seaweed products prevented these disorders and in time, it was found that the missing nutrient was iodine. Now iodides (salts of iodine) are added to table salt and iodine deficiency is rare. A diet that includes occasional ocean fish or the taking of kelp concentrate easily meets one's iodine requirements. If one were to avoid iodized salt, I would recommend daily kelp concentrate for its iodine content. Paradoxically, excessive iodine intake can also lead to goiter.

Chapter 12

HORMONE BALANCE
AND OSTEOPOROSIS

As my family practice got older, so did my patients. After thirty years, my thirty-year-old patients were sixty and my fifty-year-old patients were eighty. The many women coming to my office debilitated from osteoporosis was one of my biggest inspirations to begin researching ways to prevent and reverse this distressing disease. I noticed that while calcium supplements, estrogen, and exercise seemed to make the disease less severe, they didn't prevent or reverse it. My research confirmed this observation.

I treated a woman who broke her arm lifting a grocery bag and another who broke a rib coughing. I watched helplessly as straight spines became hunchbacks and formerly active women shuffled along on walkers and canes. I saw evidence on X rays of the vertebrae in the spine crumbling and attended the funerals of women who had been killed by the inactivity forced on them by a hip fracture.

Osteoporosis is the disease American women are most likely to develop as they age. It is the most common metabolic bone disease in the United States: Over 45 percent of white women age 50 or more have bone mineral density over two standard deviations (SD) below the mean of normal young women. The lifetime risk of fracturing a hip, spine, or forearm is 40 percent for white women in the United States. Osteoporosis annually causes over 1.5 million fractures at an estimated cost of over $10 billion. The personal cost in quality and quantity of life is incalculable. Twenty percent of the women who fracture their hip die within a year. Unfortunately, proper treatment of this dangerous and (as it turns out) easily preventable disease has been drowned in a flood of misinformation brought to you by your friendly pharmaceutical companies. Let's debunk three osteoporosis myths right away, and I'll explain them in detail later in the chapter.

DEBUNKING THE OSTEOPOROSIS MYTHS

Osteoporosis Myth #1:
Osteoporosis is a calcium deficiency disease

Most women with osteoporosis are getting plenty of calcium in their diet. It is quite easy to get the minimum daily requirement of calcium in even a relatively poor diet. The truth is that osteoporosis is a disease of excessive calcium *loss* caused by many factors. In osteoporosis, calcium is being lost from the bones faster than it is being added, regardless of how much calcium a woman consumes.

Osteoporosis Myth #2:
Osteoporosis is an estrogen deficiency disease

Not even basic medical texts agree with this—it is a fabrication of the pharmaceutical industry with no scientific evidence to support it. Osteoporosis begins long before estrogen levels fall and accelerates for a few years at menopause. Taking estrogen can *slow* bone loss for those few years, but its effect wears off within a few years after menopause. Estrogen cannot rebuild new bone.

Osteoporosis Myth #3:
Osteoporosis is a disease of menopause

This is at least a decade short of the truth. Osteoporosis begins anywhere from five to 20 years prior to menopause, when estrogen levels are still high. Osteoporosis accelerates at menopause, or when a woman's ovaries are surgically removed or become nonfunctional, such as can happen after hysterectomy. I shudder to think how many thousands or even millions of women have been doomed to a crippled old age and early death because their uterus and/or ovaries were unnecessarily removed before menopause and progesterone replacement was ignored.

WHAT IS OSTEOPOROSIS?

Osteoporosis is a progressive disease with many factors contributing to its cause. It is a disease of excessive bone loss and decreased bone density; that is, over time there is less bone, and what is left is lighter and more porous. The danger in osteoporosis is an increased risk of bone fractures, which can be painful and debilitating enough to lead to premature death.

The most common fractures occurring as a result of osteoporosis are of the spinal vertebrae, forearm, hip, shoulder (humerus), and ribs, with hip fracture the most costly and most likely to be disabling. Osteoporosis occurs earlier and with greater severity in white women of Northern European extraction who are relatively thin. It is also more common among those who smoke cigarettes, are underexercised, deficient in vitamin D, calcium, or magnesium, and in those whose diet is meat-based rather than vegetable- and whole-grain-based. Alcoholism is also a potent risk factor.

A BIT ABOUT HOW BONES ARE BUILT

Bones are living tissue and, unlike teeth, they can grow as the body grows, mend when broken, and continually renew themselves throughout life. Bone can be thought of as mineralized cartilage. The skeleton begins developing early in fetal life and grows under the influence of pituitary growth hormone until puberty, when the gonadal (sex) hormones come into play. Our bones allow us to operate in gravity by supporting our weight. Muscles attached to bone allow movement by imposing the force of torsion when we lift heavy objects or move against resistance. Thus bones are designed for compression strength (weight/force) and tensile strength (lengthwise pressure and force).

There are two types of bone cells important to the process of osteoporosis: osteo*clasts* and osteo*blasts*. Osteoclast cells continually travel through bone tissue looking for older bone in need of renewal. They dissolve or resorb the old bone, leaving tiny, unfilled spaces behind. Osteoblasts then move into these spaces and produce new bone. This astounding process of continual resorption (by osteoclasts) and new bone formation (by osteoblasts), called *remodeling,* is the mechanism for the remarkable repair abilities and the continuing strength of our bones.

At any stage in life, our bone status is a product of the balance between these two functions of bone resorption and new bone formation. If the two processes are in balance, bone mass and bone strength remain constant. During the years of our major skeletal growth, new bone formation dominates. After puberty, the processes are usually balanced.

Osteoporosis is bone loss as the result of relative osteoclast dominance: More bone is being resorbed than is being made anew. Decreased bone mass may also result from deficiency of a variety of other essential factors, such as calcium, vitamin D, and magnesium, and is given the generic name *osteopenia* or, in the case of vitamin D deficiency in the young, *rickets.*

The rate at which bone tissues renew themselves (called *turnover* rate) is quite remarkable. Our long bones, such as our arm bones and leg bones, are very dense and their structure provides great tensile strength for activities such as running, jumping, hammering, and pushing. The turnover time for 100 percent renewal in these long, dense bones (called *cortical* bones) is about 10 to 12 years.

Other less dense bone (called *trabecular,* meaning "little beams"), needing only compression strength, is constructed as an open meshwork of little struts, and is found mostly at the ends of long bones, in the heel bone, and in vertebral bones. The 100 percent turnover time for these bones may be only two to three years. Thus osteoporosis will show itself earlier in trabecular bone than in cortical bone. Likewise, the progression of (or the recovery from) osteoporosis will be revealed earlier in trabecular bone. This is why I suggest that bone density tests be done on trabecular bone.

OSTEOPOROSIS AND ESTROGEN

Bone mass in women is highest during their early or midthirties, after which there occurs a gradual decline until menopause, when the loss rate accelerates for three to five years and then typically continues at the rate of 1 to 1.5 percent per year. The menopausal acceleration of bone loss suggests that the decline in sex hormones is a causative factor. In the mid-1970s, estrogen replacement after oophorectomy (removal of the ovaries) was found to lessen the loss of bone mass when compared to untreated oophorectomized control patients. Estrogen's role in osteoporosis was further supported by population studies demonstrating that women treated with estrogen sustained fewer fractures than did untreated women. These studies do point to estrogen's role in bone loss, but, as a number of scientists have pointed out, the earlier studies suffer from a number of defects, including inadequate sample size, insufficient duration, and lack of precise bone density measurement technology. In addition, these studies tended to include a disproportionate number of otherwise healthy women who had undergone oophorectomy or had experienced hot flashes. It is now generally agreed, however, that estrogen therapy temporarily retards osteoporosis progression, but does not truly prevent or reverse it.

About the same time that studies were showing that estrogen could temporarily slow bone loss in osteoporotic women, it became evident that estrogen replacement therapy was not without risk. Estrogen unopposed by progesterone was found to cause salt and water retention, increase blood clotting, promote fat synthesis, oppose thyroxin (a thyroid hormone), promote uterine fibroids, promote mastodynia (breast pain) and fibrocystic breasts, increase the risk of gallstones and liver dysfunction, and, more ominously, increase the risk of endometrial cancer, pituitary tumors (prolactinoma), and probably breast cancer. It was further found that the bone benefits of estrogen replacement after menopause wane after three to five years.

Mainstream medicine strangely persists in the single-minded belief that estrogen is the mainstay of osteoporosis treatment for women. This is exceedingly odd because even the most authoritative medical textbooks do not support it, as the following examples illustrate:

- *Cecil's Textbook of Medicine,* 18th edition, 1988: "Estrogen is more effective than calcium but has significant side effects."

- *Harrison's Principles of Internal Medicine,* 12th edition, 1991: "Estrogens may decrease the rate of bone resorption, but bone formation usually does not increase and eventually decreases" and "estrogens retard bone loss ... although restoration of bone mass is minimal."
- *Scientific American*'s updated medicine text, 1991: "Estrogens decrease bone resorption" but "associated with the decrease in bone resorption is a decrease in bone formation. Therefore, estrogens should not be expected to increase bone mass." The authors also discuss estrogen side effects, including the risk of endometrial cancer, which "is increased six-fold in women who receive estrogen therapy for up to five years; the risk is increased 15-fold in long-term users."

If one pursues the supporting references for these lukewarm endorsements of estrogen replacement therapy, the evidence favoring estrogen's alleged bone benefits becomes even more clouded. None of the studies using estrogen alone showed any increase of bone mass. The modest increase of bone mass reported by Claus Christiansen et al. in *Lancet* occurred in postmenopausal women given estrogen *and* a progestin (noresthisterone acetate).

A few years ago I attended a National Osteoporosis Foundation (NOF) symposium in Seattle, where a respected researcher presented his material on estrogen and osteoporosis, including the paper referenced above. During the question period after his talk, I pointed out to him that he had given his patients both estrogen and progestin and asked him how he had concluded the benefit observed resulted solely from estrogen. After looking again at his chart he pondered a bit and then, as I recall, said, "Oh, yes, I see what you mean. That was not part of the grant protocol. But if someone would give me a grant to do such a study, I think I could find the answer." I reminded him I had done such a study, giving osteoporosis patients progesterone without estrogen, and found better bone results than his. The lesson I learned from this little exchange was that the protocols for much of the research we see published, and which parts of the outcome are emphasized and publicized as well, are determined by the grantor of the money for the research.

Since the mid-1970s, when the estrogen/endometrial cancer link was noted, all but a couple of studies of hormone supplementation in postmenopausal women for osteoporosis have included a progestin along with the estrogen. The potential confounding effect of progestins has simply never been considered.

Present evidence suggests that estrogen's actions regarding bone are only related to bone resorption. A study by Stavros C. Manolagas et al. in *Science* reported that the *lack* of estrogen stimulates production of a substance called interleukin-6, which stimulates growth of osteoclasts, thus increasing bone loss. This effect of estrogen lack causing increased bone loss is most noticeable in the five years immediately following menopause. After that period, continued use of estrogen is relatively ineffective, with bone loss proceeding at the same rate as in those not on estrogen. I would take this as an indication that, after a period of a few years, the body adjusts to the lower estrogen levels. In cultures where overall estrogen levels are much lower, and thus the drop at menopause is much less, women are less likely to suffer from osteoporosis.

The pharmaceutical industry has viewed the potential osteoporosis market as a magnificent opportunity to sell their synthetic patent medicine hormones (HRT). Doctors have been treated to massive advertising campaigns via journal advertisements, promotional symposia disguised as continuing medical education (CME courses are a requirement for physicians to stay licensed these days), personal visits by drug salesmen bringing boxes of free samples, and medical articles of studies spawned by generous grants from the industry, all touting the supposed bone benefit of estrogen and the protective effect (against endometrial cancer) of progestins. In the past few years we have been provided with reliable evidence that osteoporotic bone loss occurs in women with progesterone deficiency despite adequate estrogen levels. Yet physicians continue to be taught that "estrogen is the single most potent factor in prevention of bone loss." The strength of the estrogen fixed mindset represents a victory of advertising over science.

A 1995 issue of the *New England Journal of Medicine* reported on a major study, "Risk factors for hip fracture in white women," which was supported by no less than five different grants from the Public Health Service, involved over 9500 women in various areas of the United States, and has been eight years in the making. One of its major findings was that current estrogen use by these women over age 65 was found to have *no benefit in preventing hip fracture*! The authors, however, argue that women who had used estrogen earlier in life had fewer fractures when arriving at age 65, and thus they support the current view that estrogen protects against fracture. This very likely reflects socioeconomic differences between those who were prescribed estrogen and those who weren't, and the acknowledged benefit of using estrogen during the three- to-five-year interval around menopause time when acceleration of bone resorption *can* be slowed in United States women by estrogen supplementation. They do not comment on the fact that bone resorption after this particular time period is no longer affected by estrogen. This study showed that by seven years after menopause, the ongoing decline in bone mineral density (BMD) was the same in estrogen-treated and non-estrogen-treated women. This shows that estrogen treatment has a bone benefit only during the few years around menopause time. However, since the estrogen-treated women lost less bone during those seven menopausal years, they had a higher BMD in the subsequent years, when their yearly bone loss was unaffected by continuing estrogen treatment. The last sentence of the study's abstract (which was curiously ignored by the mainstream newspapers and magazines) says it all: "Women should take estrogen for at least seven years after menopause. Even this duration of therapy may have little residual effect on BMD among women 75 years of age or older, who have the highest risk of fracture."

These studies do not take into account the possibility of new bone formation sufficient to balance the ongoing bone loss. That is where progesterone comes in. Despite the menopausal acceleration of bone loss due to estrogen decrease, progesterone-induced new bone formation is sufficient to prevent BMD loss. In fact, women more than seven years postmenopausal will gain new bone and higher BMD from progesterone therapy whether or not they take estrogen.

If there was no other treatment for osteoporosis than estrogen, it might be worth that 10-percent savings in bone density, despite all the risks and side effects. But since my experience indicates that progesterone, combined with proper diet and exercise, steadily increases bone density regardless of age, there's no reason for any woman to have to take estrogen for osteoporosis.

OSTEOPOROSIS AND PROGESTERONE

The makers of Premarin and other estrogen manufacturers would have us all believing that estrogen loss is the major hormonal factor in osteoporosis in women. If that is so, why does significant bone loss occur during the 10 to 15 years before menopause, when estrogen levels are still normal? In the United States, it is a fact that peak bone mass in women occurs in the midthirties, and that a good percentage of women arrive at menopause with osteoporosis well under way. The more important factor in osteoporosis is the lack of progesterone, which causes a decrease in new bone formation. Adding progesterone will actively increase bone mass and density and can *reverse* osteoporosis.

Several examples illustrate progesterone's bone benefits. In 1982, a 72-year-old woman came to see me after she had fractured her arm lifting her ill husband, and had been found to have severe osteoporosis. Until then she had followed a good diet and had considered herself in good health. Her doctor had recommended a fluoride treatment, but she refused and came to me to try the progesterone skin cream therapy. After the first six months, her bone tests showed no improvement. She had been using Tagamet (a drug that suppresses secretion of gastric acid) and liquid antacids for chronic indigestion. Suspecting that her indigestion was actually due to lack of gastric acid and knowing that gastric acid is essential for calcium absorption, I had her discontinue her medications and continue with the progesterone. Soon after, she noted that her indigestion was gone (the Tagamet and antacids were no longer suppressing gastric acid secretion) and the persistent pain in her "healed" fractured arm disappeared. Subsequent bone mineral density results are pictured in the graph below.

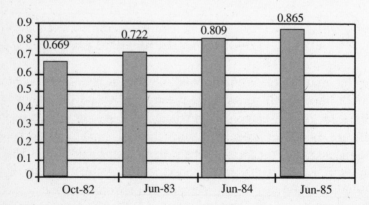

Figure 10: Serial lumbar BMD (gm/cm²) of patient, age 72, treated with transdermal progesterone

This represents a 29-percent increase in bone mineral density in less than three years of progesterone therapy. This is not at all unusual. This woman is now 85 years old and continues to do well using progesterone cream.

More recently, I received a phone call from a 72-year-old woman from Pennsylvania who had developed a very painful back due to a spinal fracture. Bone density measurements showed she had advanced osteoporosis. I had met this woman on a previous occasion at a health conference and knew she prided herself on her youthful looks, good diet, and other good health practices. She was appalled that despite all her good habits she had developed such severe osteoporosis. She had heard of my work with natural progesterone and was asking my advice. Her husband and son were both physicians. They and her own doctor told her that my ideas about progesterone and bone building were totally unsubstantiated. I sent her a copy of my treatment protocol and suggested she give it a try, under the care of her physician. Sixteen months later she sent me copies of her bone mineral density tests, performed initially after eight months and again after 16 months. They showed a progressive BMD increase of 23 percent in 16 months. Of course, she was very pleased and was happy to report that her husband, her son, her own doctor, and the radiologist were amazed, and they were all now using natural progesterone in their own practices.

Her serial bone mineral density tests follow:

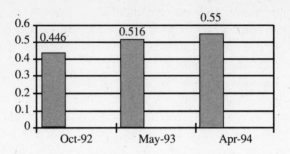

Figure 11: Serial lumbar BMD (gm/cm²) of patient, age 71, treated with trans-dermal progesterone

In preventing bone loss, we have to look as far back as a woman's early thirties. Dr. Jerilynn Prior at the University of British Columbia in Vancouver, British Columbia, Canada, measured estrogen and progesterone levels in female marathon runners who were developing osteoporosis. She found that they developed osteoporosis when their estrogen was still high. But they had stopped ovulating, a common syndrome in female athletes, and their progesterone levels had fallen. It was the lack of progesterone that brought on the osteoporosis. These women were estrogen dominant and progesterone deficient. Prior then tested nonathletic women and found a similar syndrome: In their midthirties, their progesterone levels fell. This falling off of progesterone levels due to anovulatory cycles occurs in all the industrialized countries and is epidemic in North America and Western Europe, where it is no doubt contributing to the alarming rise in infertility among women in their thirties. As noted above, osteoporosis in women typically starts in their midthirties, often fifteen years before menopause, with a bone loss rate of about 1 to 1.5 percent per year. With menopause, bone loss accelerates to 3 to 5 percent per year for five years or so, after which bone loss continues at the rate of about 1.5 percent per year. If the estrogen hypothesis of osteoporosis were true, there would be no reason for the premenopausal bone mass loss when estrogen levels remain high. Clearly there is something wrong with the estrogen hypothesis. The more important hormone is progesterone. It is during the years prior to menopause that *progesterone* levels fall due to anovulatory periods.

The accelerated loss of bone as a consequence of menopause suggests the additional effect of estrogen loss. Recall, however, that this stage of accelerated loss lasts for only four to five years, and then resumes the more typical loss rate of 1 to 1.5 percent per year, suggesting that the estrogen effect is subject to adaptive adjustment by bone cells. The following graph depicts typical bone mineral densities relative to a woman's age:

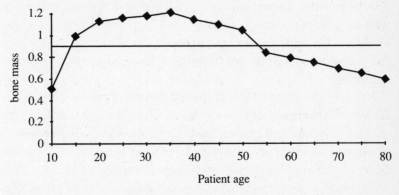

Figure 12: Schematic graph of bone mass relative to age, with menopause at age 50. Bone mass below horizontal line represents level of increased fracture risk. Note the more rapid decrease in bone mass during years around age 50—the average menopause age. Note also that bone mass loss starts a number of years before actual menopause.

On the other hand, Jerilynn Prior, M.D., has presented the evidence that progesterone does have receptors in osteoblasts, and is therefore more likely to affect new bone formation. Several small studies have further shown modest bone benefit (though less than that from natural progesterone) from the use of synthetic progestins. From the available evidence, several deductions can be made:

- Estrogen retards osteoclast-mediated bone resorption.
- Natural progesterone stimulates osteoblast-mediated new bone formation.
- Some progestins may also stimulate new bone formation to a lesser degree.

Since it is clear that estrogen can retard but not reverse osteoporosis and estrogen cannot protect against osteoporosis when progesterone is absent, the addition of natural progesterone should be used in preventing or treating postmenopausal osteoporosis. Further, since some estrogen is produced by fat cells, muscle cells, and skin in postmenopausal women, it is possible that progesterone alone is sufficient to prevent and/or reverse osteoporosis.

Between 1980 and 1989, I treated postmenopausal osteoporosis with a program of diet, mineral and vitamin supplements, modest exercise, and natural progesterone cream, which resulted in the true reversal of osteoporosis even in patients who did not use estrogen supplements. (See Figure 13 on page 165.)

A minority of the patients using transdermal natural progesterone were also given low-dose estrogen for treatment of vaginal dryness, while the majority used no estrogen. Approximately 40 percent of the progesterone-treated patients in my study had been on estrogen supplements prior to starting progesterone, and most discontinued their estrogen if not needed for vaginal dryness. Those with the lowest bone density readings at the beginning showed the greatest response to progesterone. Also, a comparison of patients younger than 70 years of age with those over 70 showed no difference in their bone response to progesterone. Further, patients who are now well up in their eighties continue to enjoy strong bones without evident bone loss while continuing their use of natural progesterone. I get regular letters and phone calls from these women telling me how well they're doing.

For example, Mary was a slim, active 70 years old when she contacted me about her osteoporosis concern. One of her great joys in life was to go skiing each winter in the Sierras with a university group in which she enjoyed being one of the oldest members. Her doctor had measured her BMD and, finding it to be low in her spine, told her she should no longer go skiing. She wisely stopped skiing and started on my osteoporosis program, including

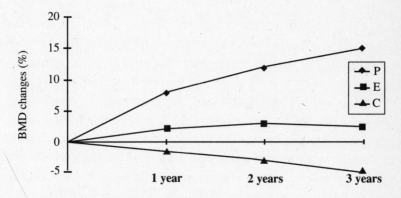

Typical BMD changes with progesterone (P),
estrogen only (E), or control (C)

Figure 13: Typical three-year bone mineral density (BMD) changes in patients using progesterone, estrogen, and controls (i.e., without hormone therapy). In this graph, it can be seen that the untreated postmenopausal patient with osteoporosis will lose 1.5 percent bone mass per year. Estrogen supplementation will tend to maintain bone mass, but only the addition of natural progesterone will increase bone mass, thus reversing the osteoporotic process.

using a natural progesterone cream. In two years her BMD had improved significantly (0.800 to 0.864 gm/cm), and she decided it was time to start skiing again! When I last heard from her she had enjoyed three injury-free ski seasons. Age is not the cause of osteoporosis; poor nutrition, lack of exercise, and progesterone deficiency are the major factors.

In 1989, when I retired from active practice, I took the opportunity to review the charts of 100 patients presently using transdermal progesterone under my care for osteoporosis prevention and/or treatment. Of these, 63 had followed through with serial bone mineral density (BMD) testing, and 62 of them had been on natural progesterone for at least three years. One patient who had gained 15 percent in BMD in less than two years was excluded because she had not yet completed three years on the program. From these records I was able to record their initial lumbar BMD results and results after three years of natural progesterone. About 40 percent of them were also using low-dose estrogen orally (Premarin, 0.3 to 0.625 milligrams daily for three weeks a month) or intravaginally for vaginal dryness. This dosage has been found in numerous studies never to reverse osteoporosis. The ages at which they had started natural progesterone ranged from 38 to 83 years, with the average (mean) age at the time of entry into the progesterone program at 65.2 years. The average time from menopause was 16 years. The majority had already experienced height loss, some by as much as five inches. The results of this collation of data follows:

Lumbar BMD gm/cm²		Initial^f	3-yr^f	net gain	% gain
0.5–0.8	12*	0.745	0.911	0.166	23.4
0.8–0.9	12*	0.838	0.992	0.154	18.1
0.9–1.0	18*	0.957	1.122	0.165	17.1
1.0–1.1	9*	1.026	1.134	0.108	10.5
1.1–1.2	8*	1.152	1.215	0.063	5.5
1.2–1.3	3*	1.256	1.289	0.033	2.6

* indicates number of patients

f indicates arithmetic mean (average)

Table 2: Three-year treatment results relative to initial lumbar BMD (in gm/cm²)

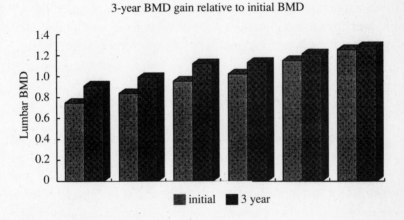

Figure 14: This graph represents the three-year improvement relative to initial BMD in the patients in Table 2.

As can be seen, women with the lowest bone densities experienced the greatest relative improvement. Those with good initial BMD either retained their good levels or improved only slightly. In these women, neither age nor time from menopause was an apparent factor. The improvement of those patients over 70 years of age was equal to those less than 70 years.

As the reader might anticipate, with experiences such as these in patient after patient over a 10-year period, I cannot doubt that natural progesterone, along with a program of diet, a few vitamin and mineral supplements, and modest exercise will effectively, inexpensively, and safely reverse osteoporosis in women. Since bone cells are not inherently different between the sexes, I would predict that the same benefits would occur in men lacking testosterone. Men with a lack of testosterone, such as men castrated either surgically or chemically, will experience accelerated osteoporosis within two to three years. Such a condition happens, for instance, in the treatment of prostate cancer. Since there is no evidence that progesterone is a risk for men with prostate cancer, I would hope that a clinical trial of progesterone would be offered to protect their bones in conditions of testosterone deficiency.

OTHER OSTEOPOROSIS TREATMENTS

The pharmaceutical industry has come up with a variety of drugs to treat osteoporosis, which predictably have limited effectiveness and unpleasant side effects. Etidronate (Didronel) and other bi- (or di-) phosphonates are drugs that slow bone loss, leading to gradual (in two years or so of use) retention of old bone and an apparent modest increase in bone mass. The accumulated old bone is, however, not good bone and results in an *increase* in hip fracture incidence by the third or fourth year of use. Bone resorption and new bone formation are linked in the sense that a decrease of bone resorption is associated with a decrease in new bone formation. In addition, bi-phosphonates are complicated to use, expensive, and their long-term toxicity is presently unknown.

Despite several requests by pharmaceutical interests, FDA approval of etidronate for osteoporosis has not been granted.

Calcitonin-salmon (Calcimar) is another so-called osteoporosis drug. In humans, calcitonin is a hormone made by the thyroid gland. However, women whose thyroid glands have been removed do not experience a higher risk of osteoporosis than women with intact thyroid glands. Osteoporosis is not a disease of calcitonin deficiency. The drug Calcimar is extracted from salmon pituitary glands. When injected into humans, there is a brief period of new bone formation. With further sets of injections, the bone response becomes progressively less. When discontinued, the benefits gained are quickly lost.

KEEPING YOUR BONES STRONG

Progesterone is not a magic bullet for curing osteoporosis. Successfully preventing and treating this disease require proper diet, weight-bearing exercise, and some vitamin and mineral supplements as a safety factor. Bone building should be considered as a chain of linked factors, each of which must be strong for the chain to be strong. Dr. Lee's Osteoporosis Treatment Program can be found summarized on page 315.

Since calcium is the predominant mineral in bone building, it is helpful to follow the chain of events that facilitate its bone use from ingestion to incorporation into bone:

Ingested calcium	Facilitating factors
↓	gastric hydrochloric acid (HCl) and vitamin D
Absorbed calcium	
↓	exercise, progesterone (stimulates osteoblasts), estrogen (restrains osteoclasts), magnesium, micronutrients. Avoid excess protein, phosphorus, diuretics, antibiotics, fluoride, and metabolic acidosis.
Bone incorporation	

Calcium

The role of calcium in bone building is widely known. When health and nutrition are in balance, one's intake of calcium should be about 0.6 to 0.8 grams or 600 to 800 milligrams daily (though it may be wise to get 1200 to 1500 milligrams if you are not a vegetarian). Approximately 98 to 99 percent of body calcium is taken up by bones, where it is used in bone mineralization and as a reservoir from which calcium can be taken to satisfy other demands, such as blood serum calcium levels, a process primarily facilitated by *parathyroid* hormone.

The source of all calcium is from earth's soil, and our best edible source is plants (broad leaf vegetables especially) that incorporate calcium into their structure along with other minerals, vitamins, and energy-rich compounds that facilitate its absorption. To be absorbed, calcium requires *both* stomach acid and vitamin D. Older folks (usually over 70) often lack sufficient gastric acid for good absorption. This can be corrected by taking betaine hydrochloride supplements with meals. The common perception, sponsored by the dairy association, is that dairy products are the primary source of calcium. Missing from this amusing perception is the fact that well over 70 percent of the people on earth live in the equatorial zone (between the tropic of Cancer and the tropic of Capricorn), where food plants grow year-round and cows' milk is not used. These people have better bones than we in the more northern industrialized areas have. Also missing from the dairy perception is the fact that cows get the calcium for their bones and milk from plants they eat.

Other factors being equal, vegetarians uniformly have better mineralized bone than people who include meat in their diet. This isn't just because vegetarians are getting lots of high-quality calcium in their diet. Meat is high in protein, and too much protein in the diet creates an excess of acidity in the body. The kidneys need to buffer the acidic protein waste products before they can be excreted in the urine. This buffering is accomplished with calcium, and if there's not enough in the bloodstream to buffer the acidic protein waste products, it will be pulled off the bone. This excessive loss of calcium creates a *negative calcium balance*. It is true that some people can adapt to high-meat diets by ingesting and absorbing more calcium to balance this urinary calcium loss, but this strategy is unnecessary if one's diet is primarily vegetarian. In the United States, contemporary medicine advocates supplementing 1200 to 1500 milligrams of calcium per day for osteoporosis prevention.

To be incorporated into bone, calcium requires enzymes, which require magnesium and vitamin B6 as cocatalysts. If magnesium and vitamin B6 are deficient, calcium is less likely to become bone and is more likely to appear as calcification of tissues and joints, leading to tendonitis, bursitis, arthritis, and bone spurs. Good bone building thus requires not only calcium but adequate magnesium and vitamin B6, in which our typical diet is deficient.

If calcium supplementation is indicated, one should know that not all calcium supplements are equal. One study using calcium citrate evaluated 24-hour urine aluminum and lead excretion, plasma aluminum levels, and whole blood lead levels in 30 healthy women. The levels were tested before and during treatment with calcium citrate at 800 milligrams of elemental calcium per day. During calcium citrate therapy, urinary aluminum excretion and plasma aluminum levels increased significantly. There were no changes in urine or whole blood lead levels. The authors conclude that calcium citrate significantly increases absorption of aluminum from dietary sources. The long-term effects of calcium citrate supplementation need to be assessed. Calcium carbonate is the least expensive but also the least well absorbed. This is relatively unimportant because higher doses can be easily used. Calcium citrate is more expensive, but results in better calcium absorption when stomach acid is low. Thus it may be preferred if you are over 50.

Phosphorus

After calcium, phosphorus is the second most prevalent mineral in bones. Bone experts regard an ideal phosphorus/calcium intake ratio to be below 1.5:1. Excess phosphorus intake causes an imbalance of this ratio, leading to *decrease* in bone calcium.

Parathyroid hormone (PTH) primarily controls calcium levels in your blood. Low calcium levels trigger the release of PTH, which acts in a complex manner on three main organs (intestine, bone, and kidney) to restore calcium levels. PTH causes calcium release from bone, inhibits absorption of inorganic phosphorus by the kidneys, and, with vitamin D, increases absorption of calcium.

In bone formation, the proper ratio of phosphorus and calcium is important. If phosphorus is high relative to calcium, PTH causes osteoclasts to increase in size, number, and activity, leading to enhanced osteoclast activity and bone resorption (i.e., you lose bone). This action is dependent on nearby osteoblasts, which are the primary targets for PTH, as osteoclasts contain no PTH receptors. PTH triggers osteoblasts to release local effectors (possibly interleukin 1 or a prostaglandin), which serve to stimulate osteoclasts to resorb bone. Thus, even though phosphorus is needed by bones, an excess of phosphorus relative to calcium can actually lead to bone loss. Since the typical U.S. diet is in fact high in phosphorus, its supplementation is not indicated. Sodas—any artificially carbonated beverages—are high in phosphorus, as is red meat, and both should be restricted.

Magnesium

Magnesium, the third most prevalent mineral in bones, not only *increases* calcium absorption but facilitates its role in bone mineralization. Magnesium deficiency is common in the United States, due to our food-growing techniques, our food processing, and our diet choices. This important mineral is normally abundant in nuts, seeds, whole grains, and vegetables of all sorts, the diet of our ancestors. Our grains, originally high in magnesium, are "refined," a process that removes the outer fibrous coat along with its magnesium, zinc, and other minerals. We eat more meat (low in magnesium) and dairy products (with a poor magnesium to calcium ratio). Our use of fertilizer that contains large amounts of potassium, a magnesium antagonist, results in foods lower in magnesium than ever before. Further, sugar and alcohol consumption will both increase urinary excretion of magnesium, leading to magnesium deficiency. Interestingly, chocolate is high in magnesium. Chocolate craving can be a sign of magnesium deficiency, and this craving will often fade when magnesium intake is raised to adequate levels.

As described above, magnesium deficiency impairs utilization of calcium for bone building and results in calcium deposits in soft tissue rather than bone. In magnesium deficiency, calcium deficiency develops despite supposedly adequate supplementation. When adequate magnesium is supplied, calcium levels also rise, even without calcium supplementation. Thus proper dietary choices and adequate magnesium supplementation are vital to healthy bones. A common supplement dose of magnesium is at least 300 milligrams per day. Magnesium should be taken in a buffered form, such as magnesium gluconate or citrate, to avoid the side effect of diarrhea, and is often combined with calcium in one tablet.

Other Bone-Building Minerals

Zinc is essential as a cocatalyst for numerous enzymes, including those that convert beta-carotene to vitamin A within cells. This is especially important in building the collagen matrix of cartilage and bone. As with magnesium, zinc is one of the minerals lost in the "refining" of grain. As a result, the typical United States diet is deficient in zinc, and modest supplementation (15 to 30 milligrams a day) is recommended.

Manganese, boron, strontium, silicon, and copper are also involved in building healthy bones. A diet of whole, unprocessed foods is usually sufficient in providing these minerals.

Vitamin D

Vitamin D is essential for calcium and phosphorus transport from the intestine into the blood plasma; it decreases excretion of calcium and phosphate from the kidneys, and it facilitates mineralization of bones. Thus it is a key player in bone building. If vitamin D is deficient in young children, bones are incompletely mineralized, and this results in enlarged wrists, ankles, and bowed legs, a condition named rickets. Although rickets was first described in 1650 by Professor Glisson of Cambridge, not until the early part of this century was rickets learned to be limited to populations that lacked either fish oils or sufficient skin exposure to sunlight.

The missing factor came to be called vitamin D, the fourth vitamin to be discovered (after A, B, and C). The same disease in adults is called osteomalacia (soft bones), or the more generic term, osteopenia (bone deficiency). If vitamin D were discovered today, it would have been called an essential hormone. It is unusual in that its synthesis in the skin requires ultraviolet light. Vitamin D deficiency is common during winter months (when more of the skin is covered by clothing) and is common among the elderly. Supplementation with 300 to 400 IU of vitamin D (cholecalciferol) is sufficient for most people. High doses of vitamin D continued over a long period are *not* recommended due to the possibility of calcium deposition in soft tissues such as synovial membranes (leading to arthritis), the kidneys, the myocardium, the pancreas, and the uterus.

Vitamin A

Vitamin A is important in the synthesis of connective tissue and the collagen matrix of cartilage and bone. It is normally produced within the cells via its precursor, beta-carotene, found in yellow and deep green vegetables such as carrots, peppers, yams, sweet potatoes, string beans, leafy greens, and many other vegetables and fruits. The metabolic conversion of beta-carotene is inefficient if insufficient zinc is present to serve as an enzyme co-catalyst. The typical United States diet is deficient in zinc, due primarily to the common use of refined grain. Thus it is wise to recommend a combination of beta-carotene and zinc, with 15,000 to 25,000 IU of beta-carotene and 5 to 15 milligrams of zinc.

Vitamin C (ascorbic acid)

This vitamin is essential to the synthesis and repair of all collagen, including cartilage and the matrix of bone. Throughout the animal kingdom, vitamin C is synthesized by all but a very few species—at a daily rate of about 4 grams (4000 milligrams) per

100 pounds of animal. Most of the non-vitamin-C-producing animals choose (if free to do so) a diet that provides them with that amount of vitamin C. The typical United States diet provides only about 60 milligrams of vitamin C, or 1/70 of the animal standard. Generally, an adequate supplement of vitamin C should be 1 to 2 grams (1,000 to 2,000 milligrams) per day.

Vitamin K

This valuable vitamin, necessary for normal blood clotting, is also a beneficial factor in bone building. Studies indicate vitamin K will reduce calcium excretion and will facilitate binding of osteocalcin (an important bone protein) to hydroxyapatite crystal. Fortunately for most of us, our colon bacteria synthesize sufficient quantities daily under normal circumstances. Prolonged use of broad-spectrum antibiotics, however, may reduce intestinal flora such that vitamin K production is deficient for us. Such people may need supplemental vitamin K not only for maintaining normal blood clotting, but also for its benefit to bone and the prevention of osteoporosis.

Vitamin B6 (pyridoxine)

Pyridoxal-5'-phosphate, the active form of vitamin B6, is a co-catalyst along with magnesium for a large number of enzymes. As such, it is a facilitator in the production of progesterone and reduces inflammatory reactions in connective tissue and collagen repair. Several studies have found low B6 levels in osteoporosis patients relative to same-age controls. Since this vitamin is inexpensive and remarkably safe at effective levels (50 milligrams once or twice a day), it is wise to supplement it.

Exercise

Bone building responds to exercise. Immobilizing an arm in a sling for a prolonged period will result in bone mass loss in that arm. Immobilization in bed will result in bone loss throughout the skeleton. Astronauts in a so-called gravity-free (actually, gravity balanced by centrifugal force) environment will begin losing calcium within a couple of days. Mineralized bone (hydroxyapatite) is a crystalline structure and, as such, will respond to physical stress just as other crystalline structures do. In particular, any force tending to distort the crystalline arrangement generates an electric voltage, called the piezoelectric effect, producing a small electric current (discovered by Pierre Curie in 1883). This also happens in mineralized bone, and may explain the wondrous ability of osteoclast and osteoblast action in constructing and reinforcing bone trabeculae along lines best suited for maximum strength and physical efficiency. When viewed microscopically, trabeculae remind one of the vaulted chambers and flying buttresses of the best Gothic cathedrals.

Our modern-day, laborsaving devices and engine-powered travel have greatly reduced the exercise previously experienced in everyday living. This lack of exercise diminishes the stimuli that promote bone strength. This, along with nutritional deficiencies, is probably the primary reason for the decrease in bone mineralization now evident. When bone mineral density is compared between present-day skeletons and those buried two centuries ago, as reported recently in *Lancet*, the "ancient" bones showed better BMD results than "modern" bones. The specific form of exercise to benefit bone is relatively unimportant as long as it imposes some exercise against resistance. Exercise such as walking, bicycle riding, tennis, and weight lifting works well to build bone. Swimming is not an exercise that would build bone if done in a "lazy" fashion, but it does result in bone building if done strenuously. In otherwise healthy postmenopausal women, 22 months of weight-bearing exercise increased the density of the lumbar spine by 6.1 percent, whereas women not exercising lost bone. Bone building simply does not occur in the absence of physical stress on bones. In advanced osteoporosis, however, some care must be given to avoid excessive force that could increase the risk of fracture.

HOW BONES ARE DEPLETED

Just as attention must be paid to factors that promote good bones, so one must pay attention to factors that are deleterious to bone.

Excess Protein

Protein is essential for tissue growth and repair, and for enzyme synthesis, nucleic acids, neurotransmitters, and some hormones (e.g., insulin). For many years, science endorsed the concept of eating large amounts (120 to 185 grams a day) of protein, based on the theory of Liebig in the early nineteenth century that muscle protein is actually consumed by activity and must be constantly replaced. The fact that a large intake of protein is unnecessary was first suggested by Chittenden in 1905. However, it is only recently that science has agreed that protein requirements for adults are generally only about 40 to 60 grams (or 1.5 to 2 ounces) per day. Red meat, for example, is about 25 percent protein. Thus a six-ounce, low-fat hamburger provides 1.5 ounces of protein, meeting your recommended daily allowance. Any additional protein eaten that day may result in calcium loss. Eating meat daily in larger quantities is sure to result in calcium loss from bones and increase one's risk of osteoporosis.

If one eats more protein than required for nutritional purposes, it is not stored by the body (as fat is, for example) but must be excreted. Excess protein waste products are excreted in the urine. As we discussed earlier, the excretion of protein waste products through the kidneys increases the urinary excretion of calcium. The ratio between calcium ingested and calcium lost in urine is called the *calcium balance*. A high intake of protein creates a negative calcium balance (i.e., more is lost than was ingested). A negative calcium balance will cause it to be pulled from the bones.

In calculating protein intake, it is important to consider the protein content of various dietary components. The following list may be helpful:

Most meats ....approximately 25 percent protein

Chicken, turkey, cheese,
and fish ....25 to 30 percent protein

Beans, peas, and nuts ....approximately 10 to 12 percent
                                                     protein

Other vegetables....................range from 3.5 to 10 percent
                                                     protein

One egg (egg white)..............0.22 ounces protein; same as
                                                     one bagel

Diuretics

Diuretics increase urine volume and are used extensively in medicine to treat edema, congestive heart disease, high blood pressure, or water retention from any cause. The use of diuretics correlates with increased fracture risk. A number of diuretics cause increased urinary excretion of minerals. Furosemide (Lasix) promotes the greatest loss of calcium, thus a potential cause of osteoporosis. Other diuretics (e.g., thiazides) retain calcium, but tend also to increase one's fracture risk by causing nocturnal urination, which, among the elderly, increases the risk of accidental falls in the bathroom.

A better approach to water retention problems is by diet (avoid salty foods and sodium bicarbonate), if possible. If diuretics must be used, it is wise to choose those that do not increase calcium loss.

Antibiotics

Broad-spectrum antibiotics kill friendly intestinal bacteria that make vitamin K for us. Vitamin K is a bone-building factor. Long-term or frequent courses of antibiotics result in low vitamin K levels, and thereby interfere with bone building. Since body stores of vitamin K are small, a deficiency can develop in as little as one week. If antibiotics must be used long-term or frequently, it is wise to supplement vitamin K and replenish friendly colon bacteria such as *L. acidophilus*. Take both as long as you are taking antibiotics and for two to four weeks afterward.

Fluoride

For some years, fluoride enthusiasts claimed fluoride is good for bones. The fact is that fluoride may slightly increase the X-ray appearance of bone mass, but the resultant bone is of inferior quality and the risk of hip fracture is actually increased. This is found not only in fluoride doses used in osteoporosis "therapy" (i.e., 15 to 20 milligrams a day) but also in doses obtained in fluoridated communities (i.e., 3 to 5 milligrams a day). Fluoride is a potent enzyme inhibitor and causes pathologic changes in bone, leading to increased risk of fracture. Fluoride in all forms, including toothpastes, should be avoided by everyone.

The concentration level at which water-borne fluoride increases hip fracture risk is of great concern, because the U.S. Public Health system continues to press for fluoridation of all drinking water at a level of about 1 mg/L (ppm). This ambition of the U.S. Public Health system is not only outmoded but ill-advised, in every sense of the word. There are now eight good studies (and no good contrary ones) showing that fluoridation is associated with increased incidence of hip fractures. A recent report in *JAMA* found that hip fracture incidence among white women 65 years and older increased significantly in those communities in France with water fluoride levels over 0.11 mg/L (ppm). Throughout the world, water fluoride levels are generally less than 0.10 mg/L unless artificially raised. It would appear that humans can tolerate this low level of fluoride, but are adversely affected by drinking water with more fluoride in it.

Interestingly, it is now generally acknowledged by scientists that the supposed dental benefits of higher fluoride levels to children's teeth has been an illusion fostered by incompetent earlier fluoride studies and the misplaced zeal of fluoride promoters. The overall decrease in the rate of cavities in children is the same in nonfluoridated communities as it is in fluoridated communities, indicating that the change is probably due to better hygiene and nutrition. The fluoride used in water fluoridation is a toxic by-product of industry, particularly the phosphate fertilizer and aluminum industries, who wish to dispose of it by trickling it away in our drinking water supplies.

Metabolic Acidosis

Metabolic acidosis refers to an increase in the acidity (lower pH) of blood. It is necessary for the body to maintain blood pH within very narrow limits. As we saw in the example of excessive dietary protein (page 178), when acidity is too high, the body uses calcium to bring it back into balance. Cigarette smokers, for example, develop emphysema, or chronic obstructive pulmonary disease, leading to retained lung carbon dioxide and increased serum carbonic acid. One of the body's responses to the acidosis threat is to buffer the excess acid with calcium, usually taken from bone for the purpose.

Alcohol Abuse

Whether from specific alcohol toxicity to bone, magnesium loss, or other nutritional deficiency, osteoporosis is rampant among alcoholics. A history of more-than-modest alcohol use is a potent risk factor for osteoporosis.

Hyperthyroidism

Hyperthyroidism (excessive production of thyroid glands), especially that resulting from excessive L-thyroxin supplementation, accelerates bone resorption and thus promotes osteoporosis, presumably by stimulating osteoclast activity. Persons receiving L-thyroxin supplements should routinely be checked with thyroid tests to prevent this risk of bone loss.

Cortisone

From a molecular point of view all glucocorticoids are remarkably similar to progesterone so it is not surprising that they share some common receptor sites. In fact, progesterone and glucocorticoids compete for receptor sites in osteoblasts, the bone-building molecules. The "message" brought to the molecule by each of the two hormones is, however, quite different. The message of progesterone to the osteoblast is to stimulate new bone formation, whereas the message of glucocorticoids is to suppress that action. When glucocorticoids exceed normal production, as in Cushing's disease, osteoporosis results. Further, people placed on long-term use of large (pharmacologic) dosages of glucocorticoids will develop osteoporosis. In his book *The Safe Uses of Cortisone,* Dr.

William Jefferies did not report osteoporosis as a risk when *physiologic* dosages (the small amounts needed by the body for normal functioning) of cortisol or hydrocortisone were given to patients for over twenty years. The patentable synthetic analogs of cortisone now in vogue (e.g., prednisone, prednisolone, triamcinolone, methyl prednisolone, and dexamethasone) are considerably more potent and generally used in pharmacologic dosages: People taking these drugs over a long period of time all develop osteoporosis. It would be interesting to see whether larger doses of progesterone could prevent or reverse the osteoporosis caused by these drugs.

IN A NUTSHELL

Having summarized the various factors required for healthy, strong bones and the factors deleterious to bones, it is important that the central thesis of this chapter be restated: *Postmenopausal osteoporosis is a disease of excess bone loss caused by a progesterone deficiency and secondarily a poor diet and lack of exercise. Progesterone restores bone mass. Natural progesterone hormone is an essential factor in the prevention and proper treatment of osteoporosis.*

When all the right factors are present, bone building continues throughout life. Whenever I see a woman bent over from osteoporosis, I wish she could have been given the benefit of natural progesterone. I receive letters regularly from women with success stories. The following letters were written to me on three consecutive Christmas cards by a woman who was 81 years old at the time of writing the first letter:

Dear Dr. Lee,

Since I first wrote you [about 2-1/2 years ago], I have been using the progesterone cream every day. I found that my benefits did not peak at four months of using the cream but continued on a cumulative basis.

I can get into and out of bed without taking a few breaths to settle down and feel comfortable—I feel comfortable immediately. In the morning, I do not have to sit on the edge of the bed to adjust; I am adjusted at once. I can shift my position in bed without supporting myself at my hips.

I can walk without feeling that my back will collapse, and I can walk at a good clip! In driving I no longer need to hold myself rigid to keep from feeling that my spine is slipping at a turn, and I no longer dread any normal unevenness in the road surface.

I am able to hold saucepans of soup and carry them across the kitchen. (Previously, I had to carry an empty saucepan to the stove and then fill it cup by cup.) I can fill a quart bottle and carry it easily across the room. I can stand free and take a picture with my camera—I used to have to brace myself by leaning against a wall. I used to have to hold onto my bureau to dress and undress; now I only have to hold on for clothes I have to step into. Over the head clothes I can stand free. I can brush my teeth without having to lean on the counter.

I feel so wonderful and am so very grateful for your consideration in my regard.

One year later:

Dear Dr. Lee,

I continue to get better and better. Now I can turn my head around to back out of a parking lot. When I last wrote you my back had improved driving on turns, but now it is even more solid and I don't even think about it anymore.

Last July I flew to Boston to be with my families in five different locations with many long car trips riding with my daughter or grandaughter. I had no problem with my back and slept comfortably in five beds!

It is miraculous to have a solid back. The enclosed picture is of me and my sister, whose caretaker I am. She has considerable dementia and aphasia, but we are doing very well. I keep her as active as possible.

By the way, I can now pick things up off the floor, although I am exceedingly careful in doing so.

Sincerely and gratefully,

One year later:

Dear Dr. Lee,

All the improvements I told you about continue and more so. I can lift a ten-inch iron frying pan with one hand from the bottom shelf, and easily load and unload the dishwasher. It is wonderful to be strong and I have no pain!

Thank you! Thank you! Thank you!

MEASURING BONE MINERAL DENSITY

Any type of diagnosis or treatment program for osteoporosis should begin with a bone mineral density (BMD) measurement. That will give both you and your doctor a baseline with which to measure the results of treatment. Following the baseline measurement, BMD can be measured every two to three years thereafter to track the results of the treatment.

Aside from bone density measurements, one of the first indicators of osteoporosis is a loss of height. Women should accurately measure their height when they are 30 and then have it measured every year thereafter. Any decrease in height caused by a deterioration of the spinal bones is most likely an indicator of osteoporosis.

Prior to the 1980s, physicians lacked an accurate test of bone mineral density (BMD). Routine X ray, for example, cannot reliably measure bone mass loss or gain until the change exceeds 30 percent. We now have access to new techniques that are reliable and accurate.

Photon absorptiometry measures the decrease in energy in a photon beam passing through tissue. Photons pass easily through skin and fat, but are deflected by the minerals in bone. If you hold a flashlight up to your hand in a dark room, you can see a similar effect: Your bones make a dark shadow due to their mineral density. This method works well for the dense cortical bone found in the arms and legs.

Dual photon absorptiometry (DPA) uses photons of a slightly different absorption spectra, and is 96 to 98 percent accurate for the less dense trabecular bone found in the hips and spinal column.

Dual energy X-ray absorptiometry (DEXA) is 96 to 98 percent accurate but uses low-dose X rays.

The QCT technique, a modification of the CT or CAT scans, is also very accurate, but uses *much* more X ray and is more expensive. I don't recommend it.

Urinary excretion of pyridinium, while not a specific test for osteoporosis, can indicate rapid bone turnover rate. When bone undergoes resorption (bone loss), very specific types of pyridinum, called pyridinoline and deoxypyridinoline, are excreted in the urine. By measuring the ratio of these substances in the urine, the rate of bone turnover can be measured. Higher ratios indicate greater turnover, such as occurs in more rapid bone resorption. Since urinary excretion of the pyridiniums is also higher in cases of Paget's disease, primary hyperparathyroidism, arthritis, osteomalacia, metabolic bone disease such as hyperthyroidism, bone cancer, and alcoholic bone disease, all of these must be ruled out first. This test could be used to find osteoporosis underway earlier than BMD tests would indicate it, and would also be useful for monitoring the effect of osteoporosis treatment.

I prefer DPA or DEXA because they use much less X ray and are less expensive than QCT.

From the foregoing discussion in this chapter, I hope it is clear that the more authoritative medical references find no bone benefit from estrogen, except for the five years or so around menopause when it can slow accelerated bone loss. Before menopause and after this five-year menopausal transition, estrogen has *not* been shown to promote any bone benefit. During this five-year interval, however, the use of estrogen may be of benefit in women who experience a sharp drop in hormone levels, to prevent accelerated bone loss so they become postmenopausal with better bones. In particular, estrogen does nothing for new bone formation. That is a function of progesterone and/or testosterone.

Since osteoporosis is a function of the relative balance between "old bone" resorption and new bone formation, the accelerated menopausal-time loss of old bone can be balanced by new bone formation if progesterone is supplemented during the premenopausal phase when progesterone deficiency is common. Further studies are needed to evaluate the full protective effect of progesterone treatment during the four to five years around menopause.

Finally, I wish to emphasize that osteoporosis is a multifactorial disease and that progesterone without proper diet, nutrients, and exercise is not sufficient in and of itself to prevent or reverse osteoporosis. All factors come into play. (In Chapter 19, "The Hormone Balance Program," you will find Dr. Lee's Osteoporosis Treatment Program [page 315] with specific recommendations.) It is entirely likely that not all factors are known at this time and that future research will lead to new treatments. But at the present time, progesterone is the most important factor that is missing in the standard, mainstream approach to this most important disorder facing most women in industrialized countries today.

Chapter 13

HORMONE BALANCE AND CARDIOVASCULAR DISEASE

Estrogen is being touted by mainstream medicine as a great preventer of cardiovascular disease in women. At a recent medical symposium I heard an ob/gyn speaker claim that supplemental estrogen after menopause lowered cardiac and stroke deaths by 40 percent or more. The argument was made that heart deaths in women are very uncommon prior to menopause, that after menopause heart deaths in women adopt the male pattern, and that the difference is due to estrogen lack after menopause. This benefit of estrogen, it is claimed, results from estrogen's ability to improve a woman's lipid profile (lower total serum cholesterol and higher HDL cholesterol levels). HDL cholesterol is known to protect against coronary heart disease. This neat argument has women clamoring for estrogen supplementation. But is it really true?

DEBUNKING ANOTHER ESTROGEN MYTH

I'm going to give you a rather technical and detailed critique of the Nurses' Questionnaire Study, because it is the cornerstone of proof for estrogen's alleged cardiovascular benefits. I want you to understand how easily statistics are manipulated, and how much media hype and advertising can be created around flimsy evidence. I'm also very aware that most mainstream doctors are pushing HRT very hard, largely based on this study. I want you to know the real facts.

The primary impetus for the estrogen/heart disease claim followed the 1991 *New England Journal of Medicine* report commonly known as the Nurses' Questionnaire Study, purporting to show that postmenopausal estrogen therapy reduced the risk of dying from heart disease. In truth, this seemingly impressive study is a curious report, being long on statistical abstractions and short on clinical evidence. Its data comes from questionnaires mailed every two years from 1976 to 1986 to a large number of female nurses. In 1976, some 121,700 female nurses returned completed questionnaires. The study population was limited to postmenopausal women free of any history of cardiovascular disease or cancer during the 10 years from 1976 to 1986; 48,470 women were eventually included in the study.

The authors readily admit that more than 20 studies have been published just in the past decade addressing the question of estrogen use and the risk of coronary disease, and that the question is still highly debatable. The highly regarded Framingham Study, the only ongoing, long-term, epidemiologic study in the United States, found no coronary benefit from estrogen use. Other studies have found *increased* cardiovascular disease risk from estrogen use. In her *New England Journal of Medicine* letter to the editor, following the publication of the Nurses' Questionnaire

Study, Dr. Jerilynn Prior listed 16 references disputing the claim that estrogen provided cardiovascular benefit.

For our purposes here, we will look at only a few of the oddities of the present study. While there is no doubt that a mass of statistical data was collected from these 48,470 nurses, it is odd that such reliance was based on mere questionnaires. For instance, nutritional analysis by recall questionnaires is notoriously unreliable. Yet the authors calculated precise figures for dietary intake of saturated fat, cholesterol, polyunsaturated fat, dietary fiber, and alcohol use from these questionnaires, and then used these figures to make adjustments in risk factors for estrogen and heart disease. Who can recall their precise alcohol and dietary intake over a two-year period?

It is also well known that fat and alcohol are not the only dietary factors affecting heart disease risk. Minerals such as magnesium and potassium, and antioxidants such as vitamins E, C, beta-carotene, and selenium are significantly protective, for instance. These factors were not included in the nurses' study dietary or supplement calculations.

The total number of deaths among these nurses was 1263, which is only 2.6 percent of the total number of nurses, a very small representation from which to draw any conclusions. Of these, there were a mere 112 coronary heart disease (CHD) deaths, representing only 0.2 percent of the total number of nurses, and only 8.9 percent of the total number of deaths. Over 90 percent of the nurses' deaths were from other causes. After adjusting for age and risk factors, the authors calculated that heart death risk among "current hormone" users was 39 percent less and that for "former hormone" users it was 17 percent less, compared to "no hormone" users. However, several questions (unanswered in the paper) arise:

1. Does "hormone" use indicate just estrogen or estrogen plus a progestin?
2. What type and dose of the hormone was used? (The authors report an increased heart risk with conjugated hormone use over 1.25 milligram per day.)
3. How long did the "former hormone" users use the hormones, and why did they quit? Does a three- to six-month period of hormone use qualify?
4. How long have the "current hormone" users been using the hormone?
5. On what basis did any given nurse decide to use or not use hormones?

This last question is of particular importance. Nurses are relatively well educated about the use of hormones. Did their doctors tell them not to use hormones because of some estrogen risk or contraindication, or did they themselves feel no need to even ask their doctors about it? Table 1 of the report indicates that the prior use of oral contraceptives was 42 percent higher among current hormone users than among nonusers. Why should this be? Does it indicate a significant difference in inherent or behavioral factors that might have an effect on heart disease risk?

Table 1 in the paper also indicates that cigarette smoking was 29.5 percent higher among nonusers than among current hormone users, and diabetes incidence was 29.6 percent higher among nonusers than among current users, both very potent risk factors for heart disease. Contrary to what one would think, high serum cholesterol was less common among nonusers, and no explanation is offered. Further, the current users were more likely to be lean and to engage in regular, vigorous exercise, both potent protectors against heart disease.

The following graph illustrates the difference in various coronary risk factors comparing non–hormone users and current hormone users, using data from Table 1 of the report:

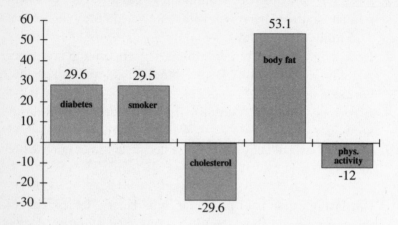

Figure 15: Percent differences in coronary risk factors, comparing hormone nonusers to current users.

Nurses in this study not using hormones were more likely to be diabetic, to be cigarette smokers, to have more body fat, and to do less exercise than nurses using hormones. Paradoxically, the nonusers were found to have lower cholesterol levels. Being fatter, were they dieting more and thereby lowering their cholesterol levels? Does hormone use increase cholesterol? Do users differ from nonusers in some metabolic way? Given all these known risk factors for heart disease among the nonusers, why do the authors implicate estrogen use per se as the factor causing fewer heart attacks? They argue that they have "adjusted" for these differences, but how did they arrive at their adjustment? A minor difference in the adjustment calculation can make a major difference in the outcome results. The answers to these and many other important questions remain unknown.

We must also question the value of risk ratios based on only 0.2

percent heart mortality among the total group of nurses. That's the equivalent of observing 500 nurses until just one dies of a heart attack. To illustrate how tiny that percentage is, we need a large pie graph. The following graph pictures the relative proportion of total deaths and coronary heart disease deaths compared to the total number of nurses in the study:

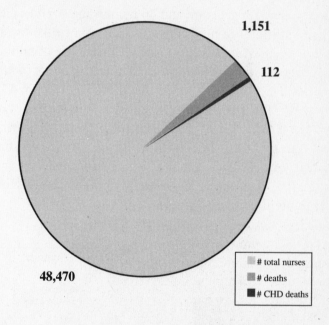

Figure 16: Deaths and CHD deaths in the Nurses' Questionnaire Study.

Notice how tiny the CHD deaths segment is, relative to the total number of nurses in the study. Is it reasonable to presume that the 112 coronary heart deaths, representing only 0.2 percent of the nurses, is of sufficient size to predict that the outcomes pertaining to "no hormone," "current hormone," and "former hormone" users will follow the same pattern among the remaining 47,207 nurses? Who can predict the hormone use distribution among the next 112 (or the next 500) nurses to die of coronary heart disease?

Finally, we should look at estrogen's risk regarding strokes. In general, strokes are of two kinds: ischemic or thromboembolic (caused by blood clots in brain arteries) and hemorrhagic (caused by bleeding from a brain artery). Of the two types, ischemic strokes are more common. Table 2 of the study shows there were 113 ischemic and 36 hemorrhagic strokes identified. The big difference here concerns ischemic stroke incidence between nonusers and current users. Current use of hormones was associated with an *increased* ischemic stroke risk of 46 percent, and with a decreased hemorrhagic stroke risk of 47 percent. However, the total number of hemorrhagic strokes is only one-third of the number of ischemic strokes. Thus it is clear that current estrogen use is associated with more strokes. Yet the authors state that current estrogen use "is not associated with any change in the risk of stroke." This is simply not the case, as the following figure illustrates:

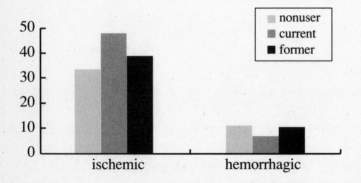

Figure 17: Relative risk of ischemic and hemorrhagic stroke relative to hormone use.

It is clear from the chart that the increased risk of ischemic stroke among current and former users of hormones is considerably greater than the modest decreased risk of hemorrhagic stroke found among current hormone users. Recall that estrogen induces increased coagulability of blood, reducing perhaps the risk of hemorrhagic stroke but increasing the risk of ischemic stroke, as was found in this study.

Despite the faulty nature of this study, it has become the cornerstone of the recent marketing campaign to convince women to take estrogen to prevent heart disease. As is the custom in U.S. mainstream medicine, doctors have been bombarded with advertisements of the claimed benefit of estrogen (with the stroke risks completely ignored). Estrogen sales zoomed. The advertisers rightly know that the typical doctor rarely reads the whole article and follows the lead of the drug sales representatives. None of the more recent studies purporting to show the heart benefits of estrogen have been any more convincing. Just for starters, most of them used estrogen plus a progestin. And, yes, estrogen does lower total cholesterol and raise the good HDL cholesterol (though not shown by the study), but at what cost? This is only one risk factor for heart disease, and a questionable one at that. Given the risks and side effects of estrogen, wouldn't it be more sensible to improve cholesterol levels through the well-proven and safer route of a good diet, exercise, and antioxidant supplements?

OTHER FACTORS IN HEART DISEASE

Given the fact that heart deaths are rare before menopause and increase substantially after menopause, what factor(s) other than estrogen lack might explain this? Dietary factors are extremely important in heart disease. The list is a long one: over-eating in general, animal fat, sugar and refined carbohydrates, overprocessed foods, excess salt or sodium, transfatty acids, lack of fiber, magnesium and/or potassium deficiency, and lack of antioxidant-rich foods or supplements such as vitamins C, E, A, beta-carotene, and selenium.

Stress is also a risk factor for heart deaths. Unfortunately, much depends on the specific type or form of the stress, as well as the manner in which stress is dealt with. The type A personality won't handle stress as well as a type B personality. These factors, too, are difficult to evaluate on the basis of a questionnaire. Nurses' stress situations vary widely, as one might imagine. Intensive care nurses burn out more frequently than pediatric nurses; night duty is different from day duty; emergency room duty is different from general care duty. When the difference in deaths is a matter of only a relatively few cases, stress differences may play an important role in the results.

Another factor in postmenopausal heart disease is iron overload. Iron is a peculiar mineral for a variety of reasons. Excesses are not excreted by the kidney as many other minerals are. The body, in fact, has no mechanism for excreting excess iron. Iron is particularly apt to initiate oxidizing events throughout the body, generating destructive free radicals. The chief cause of coronary heart disease is not cholesterol per se, but oxidized cholesterol. Anything that increases cholesterol oxidation increases one's risk of coronary heart disease. Menstruating women generally have lower levels of iron due to their monthly bleeding periods. After menopause, this no longer pertains. It is known that the disease hemochromatosis, which results in excess iron absorption, is associated with increased incidence of heart disease. Lower iron levels (and less coronary heart disease) may simply be one of the benefits of menstruation.

PROGESTERONE AND CHOLESTEROL

What about progesterone? We now know that anovulatory cycles and lowered progesterone levels occur prior to menopause, and progesterone levels after menopause are close to zero. Estrogen, on the other hand, falls only 40 to 60 percent with menopause. A woman's passage through menopause results in a greater loss of progesterone than of estrogen. Perhaps the increase in heart disease risk after menopause is due more to progesterone deficiency than to estrogen deficiency. In my clinical experience, lipid profiles improve when progesterone is supplemented. In the PEPI study, lipid profiles in women on combined HRT were considerably better in women receiving natural progesterone than in those receiving the progestin medroxyprogesterone acetate.

Progesterone increases the burning of fats for energy and, in addition, has anti-inflammatory effects. Both of these actions would be protective against coronary heart disease. Progesterone protects the integrity and function of cell membranes, whereas estrogen allows an influx of sodium and water while allowing loss of potassium and magnesium. Progesterone, a natural diuretic, promotes better sleep patterns and helps one deal with stress. When one reviews the known actions of progesterone, it is clear that many of its actions are also beneficial to the heart.

The time has come to compare the heart history of the many women now who are using natural progesterone during their postmenopausal years with women on estrogen and non–hormone users. It is my firm conviction that such a comparison will reveal better results than found with estrogen alone or with added progestins.

HOW TO PREVENT CARDIOVASCULAR DISEASE

We now know a great deal about how to prevent cardiovascular disease. Although this subject will be covered in detail at the end of the book, let's briefly review what we know: We must eat less red meat and cows' milk; we must choose a diet high in fresh, unprocessed plant foods of all sorts (legumes, whole grains, leafy vegetables, and fruits); and we must restrict our vegetable oils to those with less processing and more linoleic acid and alpha-linoleic acids (like olive oil), and avoid those with transfatty acids (such as most of the others arrayed on our supermarket shelves). Contrary to common perception, eggs are not correlated with increased heart disease risk and are in fact highly nutritious. Moderate alcohol consumption has repeatedly been found to be beneficial to the heart. (Since alcohol stresses the liver, that negative effect will outweigh the heart benefits if your liver isn't healthy.)

Further, we would be wise to supplement our diet with more antioxidants, such as vitamin E, vitamin A, vitamin C, beta-carotene, zinc, selenium, bioflavonoids, and magnesium. It is well established that the protective level of these nutrients exceeds that which can be attained through normal dietary intake alone. Such supplements are safe to take and offer at least as great a benefit as that advertised for estrogen.

The medical references supporting the benefits of antioxidants are remarkably extensive. For example, there are literally hundreds of studies showing the benefits of vitamin E. If your doctor is unaware of these references, I recommend he/she study the "Vitamin E Research Summary" published in January 1993 by VERIS, which can be obtained free of charge by contacting Sharon Landvik, MS, RD, Manager, Vitamin E Research and Information Service (VERIS), 5325 South Ninth Avenue, La-

Grange, Illinois 60525. Perhaps this will inspire your doctor to seek out the appropriate references on other nutritional factors.

If the dietary advice as described briefly above (and detailed in later chapters) were followed by women, the results in protecting against heart disease (and many other illnesses, for that matter) would far exceed estrogen's supposed heart benefits. It is a dangerous fallacy to propose estrogen supplementation for all women, particularly overweight women whose estrogen production remains relatively high after menopause, merely on the basis of faulty studies such as the nurses' study. Why would a doctor want to impose upon his/her patient an increased risk of breast cancer, endometrial cancer, hypertension, depression, or loss of libido when the cardiovascular protection the patient seeks is available from safer and more effective choices? Cardiovascular disease is a big problem in our society, but adding estrogen where it is not needed is not the answer to the problem.

Chapter 14

HORMONE BALANCE AND CANCER

The use of natural progesterone by women who need it could greatly reduce the epidemic of breast cancer in Western industrialized countries. Breast cancer and endometrial cancer both occur in tissues sensitive to hormones made by the ovaries (estrogens and progesterone). Unopposed estrogens are the only known cause of endometrial cancer, though there may well be other factors involved. One or more of the estrogens are known to contribute to breast cancer incidence. Given the strong associations between estrogens and these cancers, it will become apparent as this chapter unfolds that progesterone, the other hormone made by the ovary, has a balancing or opposing role to estrogens in cancer.

REESTABLISHING CELLULAR COMMUNICATION

In general, cancer is the abnormal growth of cells in our bodies sufficient to kill us if left untreated. If we look at the big picture, cancer comes about from an imbalance in the body. Correct the imbalance and the cancer often goes away. When we focus in on the specific mechanisms of cancer, the picture becomes fuzzier. The truth is, even after the billions of dollars spent on research over many decades, we still don't understand exactly what cancer is.

The average person thinks of cancer as a foreign growth that has to be cut out, burned out, or destroyed by chemicals. This is a misguided approach. All cancer originates as a minor change in one of your own cells. Something has gone out of balance and is multiplying at a slightly increased rate; it isn't differentiating into the type of cell it was designed to be. A cancer cell *increases* its rate of multiplication and *loses* its ability to differentiate. Cells normally replicate themselves continually as needed for normal growth and repair. Each cell (with the exception of ova and sperm) contains a full complement of chromosomes, yet each develops in a manner specific for its purpose in the body. When it becomes a cancer cell, it multiplies faster than it should and loses normal differentiation. In that sense it becomes a more primitive cell, growing at its own "undisciplined" rate. These cell changes are symptoms of disease, symptoms of an imbalance. In an article in *Lancet* published in 1994, Dr. Alan B. Astrow states that, after a 25-year war on cancer, with a growing assortment of anticancer drugs, ever-more radical treatment strategies, spectacular advances in our understanding of the molecular mechanism, and so on, more and more people are dying from cancer in the United States. We are losing the war on cancer using chemicals, radiation, and surgery. Astrow says a new view has to be generated. Far from being foreign invaders, cancer cells are an intimate part of ourselves, essentially normal cells in which proportionately small changes in genes have led to changes in their behavior. The treatment strategy should be to reestablish intracellular communication, the restoration of order that begins with the establishment of communication mechanisms within the cell—a rebalancing.

HOW CANCER DEVELOPS

The actual mechanisms by which cancer begins are still speculative. There are two competing but not mutually exclusive theories. One *genetic* theory proposes that cancer is the product of chromosomal DNA damage induced by radiation, viruses, or toxins. The body combats this damage with chromosomal repair mechanisms, but as one's life progresses, the accumulated bits of damage increase over time. Thus the incidence of cancer increases with age. Factors that interfere with or impede repair mechanisms, such as toxins and stress, will predispose one to cancer.

A more recent *epigenetic* (meaning "the action of the environment") theory holds that toxic environments within the cell can stimulate an otherwise undamaged chromosome to switch to a more primitive mode of survival in response to the toxic threat. The more primitive survival mode includes an increased rate of multiplication. The epigenetic theory suggests that maintaining a healthy intracellular environment will prevent cancer, and that correcting a toxic intracellular environment may lead to successful nontoxic treatment for cancer. Evidence against the genetic theory and/or favoring the epigenetic theory includes the following:

- Under the same risk exposure, only some people develop cancer.
- Under similar exposure to known carcinogens, different individuals develop cancer at different tissue sites.
- In humans and other animals exposed to known carcino-

gens, cancer can be prevented by agents such as beta-carotene or vitamin C, which aid in the repair and maintenance
of cells.

- In cell culture tests, cancer induced by known carcinogens can be reversed and eliminated by improving the
nutrient quality of the cell culture.
- In humans with advanced cancer, survival time can often
be increased by high-dose vitamin C.
- Changes in patient attitude seem to extend survival time.
We now know without a doubt that a negative state of
mind can adversely affect the body down to the cellular
level.
- In humans, "spontaneous" remissions and apparent cures
can result from dietary changes or a combination of a positive attitude and diet.

It is common in cancer circles to separate cancer causation into
two phases: initiator and promoter. It is agreed that under normal,
healthy conditions, the chromosomes (DNA) of cells that divide
are blessed with gene segments (genomes) that repair DNA damage as it occurs. DNA damage can result from ionizing radiation,
viral attack, or chemical toxins, or it may occur at the time of early
embryo formation. These are all initiators. The defect may lie dor-
mant for years. As time proceeds, our cells may be exposed to
chemical or biological agents that act to promote cell division and
abnormal proliferation. Such agents may damage cell membranes, activate cell receptors, inactivate receptors that moderate
cell division, or may affect previously damaged chromosomes directly. All of these factors can promote cell multiplication out of
synchrony with similar unaffected cells. These agents would be
called promoters. The risk of exposure to both initiators and promoters increases as we age. Thus the appearance or manifestation

of cancer generally increases with age. Cells that do not routinely multiply (muscle and nerve cells) rarely become cancerous.

The DES (diethylstilbestrol) scenario is illustrative. When a woman takes DES during pregnancy, it causes damage to the DNA of the developing embryo/fetus, particularly the tissues of the urogenital tract. Early in embryo life, both sexes have a common, undifferentiated urogenital tract. As the embryo grows, this tract develops (differentiates) into male and female forms, becoming the ovaries, uterus, fallopian tubes, and vagina in the female, and the testes, scrotum, and penis in the male. During this time of differentiation, the cells of the urogenital tract are particularly sensitive to the potent DES hormone, and latent damage results. Later in life, this damage shows up as organ deformities of the uterus and an increased susceptibility to cancer of the cervix and vagina. In males it can lead to undescended testes (cryptorchidism), lower sperm counts, abnormalities of the penis, and an increased susceptibility to prostate cancer. Some of these effects may not manifest until late in life. The damage wrought by DES (a xenoestrogen) is not evident until late in the generation following the one exposed to DES.

From this example, we see that the timing of the exposure to an initiator can be very important, and the damaging results may not become evident for years or even until the next generation. In this regard, it is interesting to note that EPA and FDA toxicity tests look at actual toxicity and congenital defects, but do not routinely look for such late effects.

ESTROGEN STIMULATES CELL GROWTH

Both breast cancer and endometrial cancer tend to surface in women at a time in their lives when estrogen dominance is likely. In the case of breast cancer, consider the following observations:

- Breast cancer is more likely to occur in premenopausal women with normal or high estrogen levels and low progesterone levels. This situation may occur in early adult life in a few women but is quite common after age 35 or so when anovulatory periods tend to occur. It also occurs after menopause when women are given estrogen supplements without progesterone.

- Among premenopausal women, breast cancer recurrence or late metastases after mastectomy for breast cancer is more common when surgery had been performed during the first half of the menstrual cycle (when estrogen is the dominant hormone) than when surgery had been performed during the latter half of the menstrual cycle (when progesterone is dominant).

- Tamoxifen (a weak estrogenic compound that competes with natural estrogen at receptor sites) is commonly prescribed to women after breast cancer surgery for the purpose of preventing recurrence of their cancer.

- Pregnancy occurring before age 30 is known to have a protective effect. Progesterone is the dominant hormone during pregnancy.

- Only the first, full-term, early pregnancy conveys protection. Women having their first pregnancies before age 18 have approximately one-third the risk of women bearing the first child after age 35. Interrupted pregnancies (induced or spontaneous abortions) do not afford protection and may in fact increase the risk of breast cancer.

- Women without children are at a higher risk than those with one or more children.

- Women subjected to oophorectomy (removal of both ovaries) prior to age 40 have a significantly reduced risk of breast cancer.

- The protective effects of early oophorectomy are negated by the administration of estrogen.
- Treatment of males with estrogen (for prostatic cancer or after transsexual surgery) is associated with an increased risk of breast cancer.
- Recently, industrial pollutants having potent estrogenic effects, called *xenoestrogens,* are being recognized as a pervasive environmental threat, likely to be a contributing factor in the incidence of breast cancer. Such correlations strongly suggest that estrogen, especially if unopposed by progesterone, is somehow related to the development of breast cancer.

Estrogen's job in the uterus is to cause proliferation of the cells. Under the influence of estrogen, uterine cells multiply faster, and then progesterone normally should come on the scene with ovulation and stop the cells from multiplying. Progesterone causes the cells to mature and enter into a secretory phase that causes the maturing of the uterine lining, which is now ready to receive a possible fertilized egg. An analogy would be the growth of an apple: When it's finished growing, it begins to ripen. Estrogen is the hormone that stimulates cell proliferation, or the growing phase. Progesterone is the hormone that stops growth and stimulates ripening.

Estrogen dominance also stimulates breast tissue: Premenstrual women who are estrogen dominant often suffer from breast swelling and tenderness. Progesterone is the hormone that brings maturation; it brings the cells back into balance, and thus can eliminate breast tenderness.

We have an epidemic of breast cancer and cancer of the uterus in the United States. We have evidence that breast cancer occurs most often at the stage in your life when estrogen is dominant for the full month and progesterone is not coming in at the halfway point at ovulation time. Dr. Graham Colditz of Harvard maintains that unopposed estrogen is responsible for 30 to 35 percent of the breast cancers. I would put that number even higher.

THE CANCER-PROTECTIVE BENEFITS OF PROGESTERONE

The cancer-protective benefit of progesterone is clearly indicated by a beautiful prospective study done by Johns Hopkins Medical School and published in the *American Journal of Epidemiology* in 1981. How would you test the cancer protection of progesterone? One good way would be to measure women's estrogen and progesterone levels, and then divide them into two groups: one with normal progesterone levels and one with low progesterone levels.

You take 20 years to accumulate enough people, and then you follow them for another 20 years to see what happens. Johns Hopkins Private Obstetrics and Gynecology Clinic did just that, and reported the results in the *American Journal of Epidemiology*. When the low progesterone group was compared to the normal progesterone group, it was found that the occurrence of breast cancer was 5.4 times greater in the women in the low progesterone group. That is, the incidence of breast cancer in the low progesterone group was over 80 percent greater than that in the normal progesterone group. This difference was not explained by when a woman began menstruating, when she reached menopause, her history of oral contraceptive use, her history of benign breast disease, or her age of first birth of child: No other factor dislodged this ratio of 5.4 times more breast cancer in the low progesterone group. When the study looked at the low progesterone group for *all* types of cancer, they found that women in the *low* progesterone group experienced a tenfold increase from all malignant cancers, compared to the normal progesterone group. This would suggest that having a normal level of progesterone protected women from nine-tenths of all cancers that might otherwise have occurred. And of course this study was published and disappeared without a ripple—there was no money to pursue the obvious implication that progesterone deficiency plays a major role in cancer.

In a 1995 study published in the journal *Fertility and Sterility*, researchers did a double-blind randomized study examining the use of topical natural progesterone (cream) and/or topical estrogen in regard to breast duct cell growth. Forty premenopausal women scheduled to have breast surgery for removal of a presumably benign lump were studied. They were divided into four groups and asked to apply a gel to their breasts daily for 10 to 13 days before surgery. One group received a placebo, one group received progesterone, one group received estrogen (estradiol), and one group received a combination of progesterone and estrogen. Blood tests were taken the day of surgery, and breast tissue taken during surgery was tested for hormone levels and the rate of cell growth. The women using progesterone had dramatically reduced cell multiplication rates compared to the women using either the placebo or the estrogen. The women using only estrogen had significantly higher cell multiplication rates than any of the other groups. The women using a combination of progesterone and estrogen were closer to the placebo group.

This exciting study provides some of the first direct evidence that both estradiol and progesterone are well absorbed through the skin, that 10 to 13 days of transdermal (on the skin) hormone application significantly increases the concentration of hormone levels in breast cells, that estradiol significantly increases breast cell hyperplasia (increased cell growth), and that progesterone impressively decreases cell proliferation rates, even when estrogen is also supplemented.

Since duct cell hyperplasia (an increased rate of cell growth in breast duct cells) is recognized as a major risk indicator for breast cancer, it seems clear that progesterone, contrary to the synthetic progestins, is protective against breast cancer.

Because the blood tests did not reflect the increased levels of progesterone that had reached the breast cells, this study also shows that testing blood plasma levels of progesterone is not useful in measuring actual progesterone absorption. A salivary hormone test would be a more accurate reflection of progesterone absorption.

It should be recalled that not all estrogens are equivalent in their actions on breast tissue. Among the three major natural estrogens, estradiol is the most stimulating to breast tissue, estrone is second, and estriol by far the least. During pregnancy, estriol is the dominant estrogen, being produced in great quantities by the placenta, while ovarian production of estradiol and estrone are minimal. Since all estrogens compete for the same receptor sites, it is probable that sufficient estriol impedes the carcinogenic effects of estradiol and/or estrone. In a remarkable paper by Lemon et al. in a 1996 *JAMA* article, it was reported that women with breast cancer excreted 30 to 60 percent *less* estriol than noncancer controls, and that remission of cancer in patients receiving endocrine therapy occurred only in those whose estriol quotient *rose*. That is, low levels of estriol relative to estradiol and estrone correlate with increased risk of breast cancer, and higher levels of estriol from endocrine treatment correlate with remission of cancer. Further, rodent studies show that estrone and estradiol are carcinogenic for breast cancer in males or castrated females whereas estriol is not.

Thus the evidence is strong that unopposed estradiol and estrone are carcinogenic for breasts, and both progesterone and estriol, the two major hormones throughout pregnancy, are protective against breast cancer. One is left to wonder why supplementation with these two beneficial and safe hormones is not used routinely for women whenever hormone supplementation seems indicated. There should be no difficulty in measuring serum or saliva progesterone levels and urinary estriol levels to determine who might be at increased risk of breast cancer and who would benefit from supplementation. Both hormones are available in their natural form and are relatively inexpensive.

A recent review of breast cancer risk factors raises the hypothesis that estrogen plus "progesterone," rather than estrogen alone, carries a greater risk of breast cancer. However, once again, the authors use the word *progesterone* at times, but the examples cited all concerned progestins. The only exception to this was in a brief summary of hormone levels and anovulatory cycles. Despite the use of the word *progesterone* in the article's introduction, the authors' conclusion is that "the estrogen augmented by **progestogen** (i.e., synthetic progestins) hypothesis predicts that estrogen replacement therapy will increase breast cancer risk, and that the addition of a **progestogen** will increase risk further [emphasis added]." With this I agree.

Another very interesting monograph is *Connections* by Scott Somerville, concerning breast cancer and first-pregnancy abortion. In it, he describes the progressively higher levels of progesterone that occur throughout pregnancy, causing growth and permanent maturation of breast cells (milk ducts), the end result of which is not only a breast prepared for breast-feeding, but a level of maturation that makes the cells resistant to cancer changes. If this process is interrupted by the early termination of pregnancy, the breast cells remain in a transitional state more susceptible to cancer changes. Thus carrying one's first pregnancy to term protects against breast cancer. Theoretically, once a woman has a full-term pregnancy and the breast cells become fully matured, she is also protected. Thus the greatest risk factor would be for a woman who has an abortion in a first pregnancy and never carries a pregnancy to term, leaving the breast cells in an ongoing state of limbo.

BREAST CANCER

Breast cancer incidence has now risen to become the most frequently diagnosed cancer in women—175,000 cases per year, accounting for over 44,000 deaths. The incidence of breast cancer, previously the leader among women, may soon be eclipsed by lung cancer, which is rising at an even more rapid rate, an effect of increased cigarette smoking by women. The incidence of breast cancer rises with age, but is also increasing in younger, premenopausal women as well as in postmenopausal women. The incidence increases with age, such that the risk of breast cancer is now about one in 10 for women over 75 years of age. Experts agree that environmental risk factors, such as diet, account for about 80 percent of breast cancers, and genetic factors account for about 20 percent. Recently it was discovered that mutations of the gene site identified as BRCA 1 are disproportionately found in women with breast and ovarian cancer, indicating an increased susceptibility from this gene site. The number of women so afflicted may represent only a small portion of the total number of cases of breast or ovarian cancer.

Among the environmental risk factors for breast cancer, diet is probably predominant, with dietary fat being the most suspicious. Some studies report little or no association of dietary fat to breast cancer, but such studies usually err in comparing women with insufficient differences in their generally high level of fat intake; nor do they compensate for differences in the *type* of fat, the differences wrought by fat-soluble toxins such as petrochemical toxins (e.g., xenoestrogens) that may be carried by fat, or the protective effect of phytoestrogens found in plant-based diets.

The majority of studies confirm the association of dietary fat to breast cancer. These data are well presented in Dr. Robert Kradjian's book, *Save Yourself from Breast Cancer* (Berkley Books, New York, 1994). Breast cancer incidence is highest in Western (North American and Western Europe) women, where fat intake averages about 40 percent of the diet, and lowest in third-world women, where fat intake is about 15 percent of the diet. The difference in breast cancer incidence between these two populations is sixfold.

There is an inseparable connection between fat and estrogen. Breast tissues accumulate fat. Women become caught in a cycle where increased body fat raises estrogen levels, and estrogen increases the tendency to accumulate body fat. In the United States, our diet is high in animal fats, refined (transfatty acids) fats and oils, and refined carbohydrates, and low in vegetables, fruit, and fiber. In contrast, in third-world countries, diets are low in fat and high in whole, unrefined grains and vegetables. As a consequence of their higher fat consumption, United States women produce more estrogen than third-world women.

We know that estrogen increases proliferation of breast cells, but other factors relating to obesity may also increase breast cancer risk. An intracellular, insulinlike, growth factor called IGF-1 has been shown to increase human breast cancer cell replication in vitro (cell cultures). The levels of IGF-1 in a woman's body increase with insulin resistance, which is correlated with increased fat intake and body fat. Thus fat and estrogen are synergistic for increased breast cancer cell replication.

In addition, one must keep in mind that not all fats are the same. Natural fats and oils, such as olive oil (which does not require the high pressure, heat, and extensive processing of many other commercial oils), are correlated with less breast cancer than animal fats. Certain processed oils, such as margarine and the oils found in cakes, cookies, and other processed foods, contain high levels of transfatty acids as a result of the processing techniques and these are more likely to damage cell membranes and induce cancerous changes. Fats can also contain fat-soluble toxins and xeno-estrogens, which either increase cell stress or actively promote carcinogenic changes.

As described earlier, it is helpful to separate potential cancer causes into two categories. One set of factors may initiate the change of a normal cell into a cancer cell, whereas the other set may promote cancer cell growth but not initiate cancer. It is not clear whether estrogen can initiate cell changes, but it is certainly a promoter of breast cell replication. Most breast cancer cells have receptors for estrogen, and for this reason estrogen is considered a promoter of breast cancer growth.

HORMONE RECEPTORS IN BREAST CANCERS

Tests have been developed that show whether a breast cancer has receptors for estrogen and progesterone. What if the cancer tests positive for progesterone? Is that a sign that a woman shouldn't be using progesterone? Quite the opposite. One must keep in mind the "message" (effect) of the hormone. In the case of progesterone, the hormone will most likely be beneficial in helping to keep the cancer cells under control. The positive progesterone receptor test is merely a sign that the cancer is receptive to the balancing and anticancer effects of progesterone.

Hormones float through the bloodstream and the fluid around the cells, and they only work if they unite with a receptor on the cell that is already designed to be there. The hormone fits into the receptor like a lock in a key. If the receptor is there, they hook up and make their way to the celluar DNA and chromosomes, and turn on the appropriate gene site of a chromosome to produce an effect, a hormone or an action in that cell. Then, once that message has been sent, the hormone is released.

Hormones only work if the receptor site is present on the cell. When a doctor calls me and says, "Mrs. Jones has cancer and had a breast surgery, and the tests show that her cancer is progesterone positive. Should she be on progesterone?" I tell him that if she has progesterone site positive, that's the only way the progesterone could ever work! If the cancer is estrogen site positive, she should not have estrogen, because estrogen causes the cell to multiply. Progesterone causes the cancer to stop multiplying. Mrs. Jones is a perfect candidate to use progesterone.

When estrogen and progesterone receptor testing of breast cancer cells is done, it is generally the rule that progesterone receptors are not found unless plenty of estrogen receptors are present. Estrogen stimulates the emergence of progesterone receptors. Since estrogen stimulates cell proliferation (which is not desirable in cancer cells) and progesterone inhibits proliferation in favor of cell maturation, it would seem wise to supply the needed progesterone. At the present time this conclusion is a hypothesis since, to my knowledge, such research has not yet been done.

It should be recalled that the breast cancer growth rate is quite variable; the doubling time ranges from one month to over two years, with the average doubling time being about three months. Even at that relatively rapid rate of growth, it is estimated that the time from the emergence of a single cancer cell to its growth to a size sufficient for diagnosis by palpation (touch) is typically about eight to ten years (diagnosis by mammogram may be made, at most, two years earlier). This lag time between onset and diagnosis means that many breast cancers start during the 10 to 15 years before menopause,which is the premenopausal time when estrogen dominance is so common. Thus progesterone supplementation in women with low progesterone levels during these years might well be effective prevention against breast cancer.

. WHAT ABOUT MAMMOGRAMS?

Mammograms are low-energy X-ray views of breasts obtained for the purpose of detecting breast cancer earlier than by palpation, in the hope that the risk of dying from breast cancer can be reduced. While this hope may appear sensible to most, appearance and reality are not necessarily the same thing. The lag time between cancer inception and diagnosis even by mammograms may well be over eight years. Diagnosis by palpation can be made about two years later. If the cancer is one that is prone to metastasize, why would it not have metastasized during the years before the mammogram? Where is the evidence that this two-year difference in time of diagnosis will make any difference? And if a given test is found negative, how often should mammograms be repeated? If one accepts the argument that the two-year time interval between mammogram diagnosis and palpation diagnosis is crucial, to be consistent one would have to argue that, to be effective, mammograms should be performed at least every two years. Good evidence for answers for all of these questions is lacking.

Then we have the problem of reliability. Just how good are mammograms at accurately detecting breast cancer? A large Canadian study found that women utilizing mammograms experienced a higher mortality from breast cancer than women who did not have mammograms. This study was discounted by the pro-mammogram spokespeople on the basis of the quality of the mammograms done. If this argument is correct, how does a woman know whether the mammogram she had was a good one or not? It is common knowledge that 30 percent of positive readings turn out to be false and, when cancer is present, a negative reading is reached 10 to 20 percent of the time. Patricia was a trim and youthful forty-two-year-old woman who came into my office for a routine examination. As I was showing her how to do a breast self-exam, I discovered a small lump in one of her breasts. She told me she had found the lump a year before and, after several months of procrastination, had seen a doctor who ordered a mammogram, which, she was pleased to say, had been negative. She had been advised to wait a year before repeating the test. On my advice she obtained an excision biopsy of this easily palpable lump. The biopsy found breast cancer, and she decided to have a simple mastectomy. Now, ten years later, she is healthy and active. The negative initial mammogram increased her danger by delaying prompt treatment of a suspicious lump.

Recently I received a letter from a woman named Shirley, who, at age 42, detected a firm lumpiness in her left breast. During the next two years she had annual mammograms, all showing a suspicious nonspecific area of density. A surgical biopsy was performed and was said to be negative. Her doctor, for reasons unknown, placed Shirley on oral contraceptives. The lumps increased in size. A third mammogram a year later showed that the original suspicious area was still there and had become even more suspicious. Shirley then had another biopsy, which found cancer, and she underwent a mastectomy and was given a course of chemotherapy. Now, a year and a half later, her chest X ray shows suspicious nodules at the base of her left lung. She is awaiting surgical biopsy of these nodules. The odds are great that Shirley has metastases, a tragic consequence of delay wrought by overreliance on nondiagnostic mammograms and a misguided or inept surgical biopsy.

Given this state of inaccuracy in readings of such import, it should not be surprising that the typical mammogram report these days is neither a clear "yes" or "no" but a highly qualified "maybe." A perfect pair of breasts, mammogramwise, is a rare thing. The mammogram reader often reports a finding of some suspicious nature (a vague sense of localized density or perhaps some minute calcifications here and there) and suggests some concern, along with the advice to check further or obtain a repeat test at some later date. The doctor and her patient are left with uneasy choices. Should they try a needle biopsy or open excision biopsy, or merely follow along with repeat tests, and, if so, how long should she wait? If the biopsy is done and no malignancy found, does it mean that perhaps the malignancy was missed? If she opts for later reevaluation rather than biopsy, what happens to the risk of metastases if malignancy is in fact present? The patient faces unpleasant choices: unnecessary surgery versus possible increased chance of death. Chronic cancer anxiety can become her normal state of mind.

Muriel came into my office at age 50 with multiple scars on both breasts from seven different excision biopsies, all of which found dense fibrocystic breasts. She readily admitted chronic cancer anxiety. In addition, she suffered from reactive hypoglycemia. She performed breast self-exams routinely and the finding of each new lump aroused fear and trepidation because of her cysts. Now, at menopause, she wanted hormone replacement therapy. Instead of traditional HRT, I recommended physiologic dosages of progesterone without estrogen. Her breast fibrocysts disappeared within six months, her sense of energy and libido returned, her hypoglycemic episodes became a thing of the past, and her tennis game improved. Further, serial bone mineral density (BMD) tests over the subsequent ten years remained good, and her cancer anxiety faded away with the improvement in her breasts.

The efficacy of screening mammography was evaluated by a recent overview study. After analyzing 13 studies, the authors concluded that mammography offers no benefit to women under 50 years of age, but appears to reduce breast cancer mortality in women aged 50 to 74. The authors admit, however, that their study could not determine whether competent breast exam by palpation would have provided the same benefit. Several peculiarities of the study should be noted. The magnitude of the apparent mammogram benefit in women over 50 was similar regardless of the number of mammographic views, screening interval, or duration of follow-up (seven to nine years versus 10 to 12 years). That is, it did not matter whether single or double views were used, or whether the test was done yearly or every 33 months. The magnitude of the mammogram benefit in this age group is given as about 25 percent. That is, if breast cancer incidence in this age group is one case per 30 women, or 33 cases in 1000 women, it means that for every 1000 women having mammograms, 25 percent of the 33 cases of breast cancer found, or about eight women, would be less likely to die of breast cancer during the next 12 years, according to this report. My hunch is that if those same women or their physicians would perform an adequate breast self-exam for breast cancer, the results would very likely be the same. In the Canadian trial, mammography did not reduce breast cancer mortality beyond the reduction achieved by clinical examination alone.

Another explanation for the presumed benefit of mammography concerns the question of the diagnosis of duct cell "carcinoma in situ." The phrase "carcinoma in situ" implies the finding of suspicious-looking cells scattered here and there in breast tissue, and not growing as a clump or tumor-mass. At one time (prior to 1992), some pathologists used this term to indicate cells they thought might be actual cancer cells at an early stage. Since 1992, most pathologists agree that these cells do not, in fact, progress to actual cancer with any risk of true cancer. These are cases found by mammograms (and not by palpation) that resulted in breast surgery, irradiation, or chemotherapy and were counted as "cancer cures" by mammogram proponents. Since they were not true cancers, these apparent "cures" created the illusion that mammograms and early treatment were effective when, in fact, no treatment was necessary.

I believe the jury on mammograms is still out, and that women can probably achieve the same benefit by carefully examining their own breasts once a month. Nobody knows your breasts better than you do. You've lived with them for decades and know how they are supposed to feel. If you don't know, I suggest you begin getting better acquainted with them, starting today. I have had women come into my office who were able to detect breast lumps the size of a grain of rice. If you don't know how to do a breast exam, ask your doctor to show you, or ask for a brochure that describes the procedure.

TAMOXIFEN

Tamoxifen is an experimental drug being tested on women who have had breast cancer or who are at a high risk for breast cancer. It competes with estrogen for estrogen receptors, much as phytoestrogens do. Like phytoestrogens, tamoxifen has mild estrogenic properties, but is considered an antiestrogen since it inhibits the activity of regular estrogens. It has been shown to inhibit induction of rat breast cancer and has become popular among doctors as a treatment for women after surgery for breast cancer. When added to chemotherapy for women who have undergone mastectomy but with positive nodes for cancer that demonstrated positive estrogen and progesterone receptors, tamoxifen, taken orally, improved disease-free survival.

Since tamoxifen's action is to compete with one's own estrogen for estrogen receptor sites in breast tissue, and it is being strongly advised for postmenopausal women after mastectomy for breast cancer, this advice is an obvious admission that postmenopausal women still produce significant amounts of estrogen. This admission underscores the fallacy of the claim that menopause is a disease of estrogen deficiency.

The question of whether tamoxifen might help prevent breast

cancer when taken by women who are at a high risk is as yet undecided. A large study of disease-free women has been proposed but is being reevaluated in the light of evidence that tamoxifen can cause liver and eye damage.

A number of herbs and foods are known to contain phytoestrogens. The herbs tend to exhibit mildly estrogenic effects. Their benefit parallels that of tamoxifen (without the adverse side effects) in that phytoestrogens occupy estrogen receptors and are less estrogenic than those made by the body. Since it is now known that reducing calorie intake reduces estrogen levels and recent studies find 46 percent less breast cancer among women consuming more fruit and vegetables, it would seem that women interested in preventing breast cancer could make modest changes in diet and derive better and certainly safer results.

ENDOMETRIAL CANCER

The only known cause of endometrial cancer is unopposed estrogen. Here again, estradiol and estrone are the culprits. Estrogen supplements given to postmenopausal women for five years increase the risk of endometrial cancer sixfold, and longer-term use increases it 15-fold. In premenopausal women, endometrial cancer is extremely rare except during the five to ten years before menopause when estrogen dominance is common. The addition of phytoestrogens (by diet) and natural progesterone during these years has the potential to significantly reduce the incidence of endometrial cancer (as well as breast cancer, as noted above). In postmenopausal women, endometrial cancer is always a result of estrogen, especially when unopposed by progesterone or a progestin. This is why unopposed estrogen replacement therapy is so strongly contraindicated in women who have a uterus.

When estrogen is prescribed to postmenopausal women, it is

not uncommon that vaginal spotting or bleeding may occur. Given the uncertainties of the significance of vaginal bleeding at this age, the doctor usually recommends an endometrial biopsy or D and C (dilatation and curettage). A common finding is endometrial hyperplasia (areas of excessive endometrial cells) or dysplasia (suspicious-looking endometrial cells). Since many doctors believe hyperplasia and/or dysplasia are a step along the way in cancer development, this finding is hardly reassuring. Quite often, the doctor then recommends hysterectomy, believing that the uterus in postmenopausal women is a useless organ, and it is better to be safe than sorry. With the uterus out, estrogen can be resumed for all its supposed benefits. This line of reasoning is not only condescending to women, but self-serving to her doctor. In pretending to act as protector of his/her patient, he/she manages to convert a side effect of a drug he administered into a lucrative surgical operation.

Nancy, a conscientious, health-minded housewife, had been a patient of mine for many years. At menopause she had developed weight gain and some loss of energy, and was fearful of old age and osteoporosis. A gynecologist she saw at the time prescribed estrogen, which resulted in breast swelling, more weight gain, and no discernible benefit. She refused to take more estrogen. I recommended that she use a progesterone cream, which relieved her breast swelling, helped her lose weight, and brought back her energy. At my retirement, she was 61 years old and doing well on progesterone. She transferred her care to an eminent gynecologist in San Francisco. He convinced her to abandon the over-the-counter progesterone cream and resume estrogen therapy. Again she developed breast swelling, weight gain, and lethargy. Her doctor increased her estrogen dosage. She then developed vaginal spotting. This led to endometrial biopsy and a finding of hyperplasia. He indicated this was precancerous and she should see a gynecologic surgeon for a hysterectomy. In the process, her medical insurance carrier on renewing her policy increased her premiums and included a rider excluding her from any coverage for gynecologic problems. In a panic she called me about this calamitous turn of events.

I asked her to request a copy of her medical records to be sent to me. Despite written requests by herself and me, the records did not arrive. Her doctor deferred to the surgeon who performed the biopsy and was recommending the hysterectomy. After several more letters and phone calls, the information finally arrived. The pathology report indicated nothing more than estrogen-induced endometrial hyperplasia. I told her to discontinue the estrogen, resume the progesterone, and to submit to nothing more than another endometrial biopsy in three months. She accepted my advice, and three months later the biopsy report was entirely normal. I wrote a letter to her insurance carrier pointing out that no pelvic disease existed and that the previous finding was merely the result of a therapeutic misadventure. I added that there was no reason to exclude gynecologic problems from her coverage and indicated I was sending a copy of the letter and the reports to the state insurance board.

Shortly thereafter, Nancy called me to report that a new policy had arrived with full coverage and that she had discovered that the surgeon to whom her doctor had referred her was the wife of her doctor, operating (no pun intended) under her own name. She also said she had found another doctor, one who agreed that natural progesterone would be fine to use. Now, six years later, she is doing well.

This kind of scenario is being repeated with hundreds of thousands of women every year. Without casting any stones, it is difficult to resist the observation that the practice of medicine, like any other human endeavor, is not immune to self-interested manipulations and questionable secondary gains at the patient's expense. How many of the annual half-million unnecessary hysterectomies are generated by such questionable medical practices? If the doctor or his colleagues are rewarded financially by the logical consequences of women using estrogen, what impetus is there for change?

Endometrial cancer is a relatively "safe" cancer, in that it generally shows itself early by abnormal vaginal bleeding and metastasizes relatively late in its course. It can be cured if a hysterectomy is performed before the cancer metastasizes. Women treated by hysterectomy for endometrial cancer are advised, however, to avoid "hormones" forever. Like patients with a history of breast cancer, they face a future of progressive osteoporosis, vaginal atrophy, and recurrent urinary tract infections without recourse to hormonal therapy. These are the women for whom I first began prescribing natural progesterone therapy. Not only did progesterone reverse their osteoporosis and, in many cases, correct their vaginal atrophy, but also none, to my knowledge, have ever developed cancer of any sort. (If vaginal atrophy remains a problem, intravaginal estriol would be the treatment of choice.) Further, among those with intact uteri, none have ever developed any uterine problems of any kind. The evidence is overwhelming that natural progesterone is safe, and only estradiol, estrone, and the various synthetic estrogens and progestins are to be avoided to reduce one's risk of endometrial cancer.

WHY YOUR DOCTOR MAY BE POORLY INFORMED

As I describe in my book for doctors, *Natural Progesterone: The Multiple Roles of a Remarkable Hormone,* the typical doctor's medical education in medical school and throughout his practice is dominated by the medical-industrial complex. He is constantly exposed to pharmaceutical advertising; even his medical journals are often nothing more than thinly disguised advertising. A recent professional journal article concerning endome-trial cancer is a case in point. This journal, published by the American Academy of Family Physicians, is sent free of charge to all academy members. A large journal printed on glossy paper, the typical issue is 300 pages, more than half of which are med-ical ads, most of them full-page and brightly colored.

The article starts out with a table listing "risk factors for en-dometrial cancer," which includes in its entirety the following:

advanced age
obesity
diabetes mellitus
hypertension
anovulatory nulliparity
polycystic ovary disease
early menarche
late menopause
prolonged exogenous unopposed estrogen use
other cancers (i.e., cancer of the breast, colon, thyroid, ovary)
previous pelvic irradiation

Note that risk factors are not the same as causes. Risk factors are merely statistical correlations, often only markers of some undefined underlying cause. If we exclude advanced age (every-one knows that cancer risk increases with age), radiation (every-one knows that ionizing radiation of an organ increases the cancer risk of that organ), and other cancers (indicating a gen-eral cancer proclivity, probably due to embryonic or inherited gene damage), we are left with a list almost identical to the risks inherent with estrogen dominance. Early onset of menarche, late menopause, and anovulatory periods all expose women to more estrogen over the years. Estrogen dominance promotes obesity and insulin resistance, hypertension, and ovarian cysts. These can be considered likely markers of estrogen dominance.

Why don't the authors state, as many medical researchers do, that *the only known cause of endometrial cancer is estrogen* and that progesterone protects against endometrial cancer? The authors do state that "to minimize the risk of endometrial cancer that is associated with estrogen replacement therapy, progestogen should be given with the estrogen." They then admit that progestogens (progestins) cause undesirable side effects such as acne, breast tenderness, depression, irritability, and unpredictable bleeding, and advise lowering the dose or changing the type of progestin if such reactions occur. (For some reason, they seem not to be able to decide whether to refer to progesterone's synthetic analogs as progestins or progestogens. Of course, never once is progesterone mentioned.)

Is it any wonder many doctors don't know anything about natural progesterone?

TRANSCULTURAL FACTORS IN BREAST AND UTERINE CANCER

While the true incidence of breast and uterine cancer in all geographic areas of the world may not be known with complete accuracy, it is generally acknowledged that these two cancers are relatively rare in nonindustrialized countries. When individuals from these areas emigrate to industrialized cultures, their cancer rates soon rise to match the general rates of their new country. The same is true of heart disease, for example. In the case of heart disease, the change in risk follows the change in diet. Diet is probably a major risk factor in both breast and uterine cancer as well.

The Western, or industrialized, cultural diet is relatively high in meat protein and fat and high in calories compared to energy needs. The third-world, or nonindustrialized, cultural diet is relatively high in fiber and largely plant-based, thus low in animal fat, and calorie intake is often considerably lower. If one looks just at the fat factor, certain relationships between disease and fat emerge.

It is now clear that calories in excess of energy needs increase estrogen levels. When energy needs exceed calorie intake, estrogen declines, reducing fertility. When calorie intake exceeds energy needs, estrogen rises accordingly. Dr. Peter Ellison of Harvard, who has conducted worldwide assays of salivary hormone levels, believes this is the primary reason for the high estrogen levels seen in premenopausal women in industrialized cultures. The estrogen levels he found in Western women are so high in comparison to levels in women of the developing world that they should be considered abnormal. He has stated, "Only at our peril can we assume that ovarian function in the Western world is somehow a model of health."

The primary cause of our high calorie intake is the fat content of our diet. Some 40 percent of our calories come from dietary fat. Many nutritionists believe that the diet should contain only about 20 percent of its calories from fat. Excess calories = excess fats = higher estrogen levels = greater incidence of breast and uterine cancer.

Yet another difficulty with our fat intake again concerns xeno-estrogens. Our food chain is awash with estrogenic petrochemical by-products from herbicides, pesticides, plastic manufacture, solvents, and emulsifiers. In addition to being highly estrogenic, these compounds are nonbiodegradable and fat-soluble. Because of the widespread use of petrochemical products in our society, they are difficult to avoid. However, the major source of oral intake of these is by way of animal fats, particularly red meat and dairy products. In their estrogenic activity, these estrogens are considerably more potent than the estrogen made by the ovaries.

They accumulate in our fatty tissues (breast, brain, liver), cause water retention and fat deposits, and, most importantly, exhaust the number of ovarian follicles. Without ovarian follicles, progesterone cannot be made by the ovaries. In women, this translates into an increased incidence of breast and uterine cancer. Thus, not only must we be concerned about the quantity of dietary fat, but also its quality.

Other transcultural factors related to breast and uterine cancer include the following:

- The Western diet is woefully deficient in plant-based nutrients and cancer fighters such as sulforaphane, phenethyl isothiocyantate, indole-3-carbinol, flavonoids, vitamin C, folic acid, allylic sulfide, capsaicin, genistein, p-coumaric acid, chlorogenic acid, carotenes, vitamin E, and others still unknown, all of which work synergistically to protect us from cancer.

- The Western diet is deficient in fiber, which is found only in plants.

- The Western diet is deficient in phytoestrogens, weakly active plant estrogens that occupy estrogen receptors that, by competition, block out the more toxic xenoestrogens and the more potent endogenous estrogens.

- Western culture is full of laborsaving devices, thus reducing exercise and energy expenditure and creating an abnormal energetic balance.

- Western culture splinters family units and other societal support mechanisms for dealing with stress, loss, and depression, promoting alienation. All of these contribute in one way or another to increased cancer risk.

Breast and endometrial cancer, heart disease, and osteoporosis are some of the greatest fears that women face as they approach menopause. Under present circumstances, these fears are well grounded in reality. However, they need not be. When the cause of any given cancer is known, prevention becomes a reality. Lung cancer, for example, can be almost completely prevented by never smoking cigarettes. For many cancers, the cause is still unknown. However, for breast and endometrial cancer, a great deal is known about their major hormonal factors. The only mystery is, why hasn't this information permeated the halls of contemporary medicine? The carcinogenic effects of unopposed estradiol and estrone and the anticancer benefits of estriol and progesterone are well established for these two cancers.

Because of its many benefits, its great safety, and particularly its ability to oppose the carcinogenic effects of estrogens, natural progesterone deserves far more attention and application than it is generally given in the prevention and care of women's health problems today.

Chapter 15

HORMONE BALANCE AND PMS

When I was in medical school 40 years ago, there was no such thing as premenstrual syndrome (PMS). Now it's a household word in Western industrialized countries. There's no doubt that PMS exists and can make a week or so out of every month miserable for everyone involved. The symptoms tend to occur consistently a week or ten days before menstruation begins and go away shortly after. Women often report a "tidal wave" of symptoms at their onset and dread the approach of each premenstrual time of the month. A good diet and exercise help, but the root of the problem is—you guessed it—hormone imbalance. Progesterone has been wrongly accused of being the hormone responsible for PMS because it's the one that's high just before menstruation. The truth is, however, that women with PMS tend to have *lower* progesterone than normal at that time in their cycle, when progesterone is supposed to be dominant, so that estrogen is dominant instead.

WHAT IS PMS?

I've seen lists of PMS symptoms that include dozens of complaints, but the most common symptoms include several or all of the following: bloating, weight gain, headache, backaches, irritability, depression, breast swelling or tenderness, loss of libido, and fatigue. Do these symptoms sound familiar? They are also the symptoms of estrogen dominance.

But the full range of symptoms includes confusion and disorientation, intemperate judgments and decision-making, mood swings, body aches, anger and verbal abuse, lethargy alternating with increased energy, alienation, guilt (at having abused friends), lack of self-esteem, and cravings for sweets, especially for chocolate. Further, every system in the body can be affected: immune, digestive, circulatory, nervous, endocrine, and dermatologic (skin). Victims of PMS may experience any combination of the above and with all degrees of severity, from mild to overwhelming.

There are two important realities to understand about PMS. They are:

1. Yes, it is real.
2. No, you are not crazy.

There is as yet no laboratory test for PMS. Diagnosis rests on the range and monthly timing of symptoms. Since the mechanisms to explain the symptoms are unknown, the malady is correctly called a syndrome—a collection of recognizable signs and symptoms. To my mind, the hormone connection is most intriguing. It is obviously linked with the monthly hormone cycle; it never occurs prior to a year or so before menarche, and never after menopause (unless you're on HRT).

Treatment of PMS has in the past included diuretics, tranquilizers, dietary changes, aerobic exercise, psychiatric counseling, thyroid supplements, herbs, acupuncture, and vitamin and mineral supplements. While each may provide some relief, none has proved to be a panacea.

THE ROLE OF PROGESTERONE

More than a decade ago, after reading of the work of Dr. Katherina Dalton in London, who defined PMS and found success using high-dose progesterone administered as rectal suppositories, I decided to add natural progesterone cream to my treatment of patients with PMS. The results were most impressive. The majority (but not all) of these patients reported remarkable improvement in their symptoms, including the elimination of their premenstrual water retention and weight gain. I have received hundreds of phone calls and letters from women and their doctors over the past few years who report that PMS has been alleviated with the use of natural progesterone. Dr. Joel T. Hargrove of Vanderbilt University Medical Center has published results indicating a 90 percent success rate in treating PMS with oral doses of natural progesterone.

As described in previous chapters, estrogen is the dominant sex hormone during the first week after menstruation. With ovulation, progesterone levels rise to assume dominance during the two weeks preceding menstruation. Progesterone blocks many of estrogen's potential side effects. A surplus of estrogen or a deficiency of progesterone during these two weeks allows an abnormal monthlong exposure to estrogen dominance, setting the stage for the symptoms of estrogen side effects. If you want to test this for yourself, have your doctor measure your serum or saliva progesterone levels during days 18 to 25 of your cycle. Low progesterone levels undoubtedly affect hormone regulatory centers in the brain, resulting in increased production of hormones such as LH and FSH. These may also play a role in the complex symptomatology of PMS. However, for most women, simple correction of the progesterone deficiency will restore normal biofeedback and pituitary function.

PMS AND THE THYROID

It's important to note here that not all of the symptoms of PMS may be caused directly by a progesterone deficiency. Hypothyroidism, for example, may cause fatigue, headaches, and loss of libido, and thus simulate PMS. (Estrogen dominance impairs thyroid hormone activity and will simulate hypothyroidism. How do you know whether you have a progesterone deficiency or hypothyroidism? Ask your doctor to test serum thyroid levels [T3 and T4] and thyroid stimulating hormone [TSH]. Normal T3 and T4 levels with elevated TSH suggest impaired thyroid hormone activity rather than a true deficiency of thyroid hormone production. In this case, estrogen dominance is probably interfering with your thyroid function.) Adrenal exhaustion or low adrenal reserve, which I believe is epidemic among working mothers in their midthirties, can cause fatigue, unstable blood sugar, mood swings, foggy thinking, and impairment of steroid hormone synthesis; these reactions can throw sex hormones out of balance and cause PMS. Similarly, women with idiopathic (i.e., without a known cause) unstable blood sugar or hypoglycemia often experience symptoms similar to PMS and will benefit from dietary adjustments. However, it should be known that estrogen predisposes one to blood sugar imbalance, whereas progesterone enhances blood sugar control.

OTHER FACTORS IN PMS

While it is likely that a hormone imbalance directly or indirectly caused by progesterone deficiency is the major factor in the majority of PMS cases, there may also be other factors that deserve attention, especially in those cases that do not find complete relief with progesterone treatment. Nutrition plays a role. For example, when your body has finished using estrogen, it is dumped, via the liver and bile, into the intestines to be excreted. Here, fiber plays an important role in binding the estrogen and holding it for elimination. A lack of fiber in the diet can cause estrogen to be reabsorbed and recycled. Because beef cattle are often fed estrogens to fatten them up for market, eating red meat can unnaturally increase estrogen levels. Recently identified xenoestrogens may also play a role in hormone imbalance.

Stress is a well-known cause of menstrual irregularity. Many women experience PMS for the first time after going off contraceptive pills, suggesting that synthetic hormone use and the prevention of normal ovulation may leave one's ovaries less able to function normally. All factors must be considered in understanding and treating PMS, and yet the problem of normalizing hormone balance remains a key factor in proper treatment. The essential amino acid tryptophan is well known as a safe calming agent and has been reported to be of benefit in patients with PMS. (Unfortunately, tryptophan is nearly impossible to get in the United States since a contaminated batch caused illness and death in some people who used it. The removal of tryptophan from the market is a highly political issue. *Uncontaminated* tryptophan is completely safe, but competes with the new and lucrative antidepressants such as Prozac.)

Clinicians skilled in homeopathy have their share of success in treating PMS. Since I am not skilled in homeopathy, I would refer patients interested in this treatment modality to those skilled in the art. Similarly, I have talked with many patients who found benefit from herbs. Here again, I am only too happy to recommend the attention of a good herbalist for my PMS patients. The same advice pertains to acupuncture, light therapy, exercise programs, meditation, and massage. These are all modalities not in the scope of mainstream medicine, nor do I understand them well enough to make a judgment about them. Since they are relatively harmless to try, and many people report benefit from them, I see no reason not to incorporate them into a program of PMS treatment if other treatment has not provided relief.

Since PMS is such a complex issue with potentially different causes, our meager understanding of it may require further research before we truly know what is going on. The technique of doing accurate, sensitive, salivary hormone assays has been improved upon and is now available for general use. That is, with a small amount (1.5 ml or so) of one's saliva, the body level of estrogen, testosterone, or progesterone can be conveniently and inexpensively assessed. I predict this will help unravel the many strands that contribute to the problem of PMS.

Many books and reports concerning PMS lack accurate measurements of hormone levels. For example, some authors concluded that, since PMS occurs during the phase of the menstrual cycle when progesterone is usually the dominant hormone, progesterone may therefore be the "cause" of PMS. What these authors missed was the hypothesis that *lower-than-normal levels* of progesterone during this phase of the menstrual cycle may be the cause. On the basis of my clinical experience and that of other doctors, such as Dr. Hargrove, who have shown that progesterone supplements are effective in treating PMS, I predict that saliva assays for progesterone will find progesterone deficiency in a great percentage of women with PMS.

Saliva assays of corticosteroids are also available. It is entirely likely that PMS, like many other diseases, is multifactorial, and that adrenal exhaustion (or lack of adrenal reserve) is another factor in this syndrome.

My advice to women with PMS is to remind their doctors that excellent tests of salivary hormone levels are available and may help in elucidating the factors underlying their condition.

Chapter 16

NATURAL HORMONE BALANCE AND PELVIC DISORDERS

The human female pelvis is a marvel of engineering. Its tissues are sufficiently elastic and its bony arches sufficiently large for the passage of babies with heads already over 50 percent the size of an adult's. Vaginal tissue during a woman's fertile years, and especially at childbirth, is the best healing tissue of the body. Vaginal mucus secretions facilitate sexual activity, protect against infection, and promote self-cleansing. The ovaries are placed in the most protected spot of the body. The uterus, normally smaller than a fist, can accommodate a pregnancy by becoming larger than a basketball, retain muscle strength sufficient for successful delivery contractions, and return to normal within six weeks after delivery. Despite its proximity to the rectum and the possibility of coliform contamination (the dreaded *E. coli*), a healthy pelvis is remarkably resistant to infection, in spite of a monthly discharge of bloody flow that might otherwise be a culture medium par excellence.

Pelvic disorders do of course occur. Conditions such as vaginitis, urinary tract infections, endometriosis, PID (pelvic inflammatory disease), ovarian cysts, mittelschmerz, uterine fibroids, and menstrual cramps (dysmenorrhea) are among the most common. Are these disorders to be expected because of some error in Nature's plan, or do they occur because of some preventable cause? Let's take a closer look.

VAGINITIS

Vaginitis occurs more often among women taking contraceptive pills. One might argue that taking contraceptive pills implies more frequent sexual activity and therefore such women are more exposed to infectious organisms. Perhaps so, but one could also argue that contraceptive pills prevent the normal hormone-generated mucus from being produced to protect them. After all, birth control pills work by suppressing normal hormones.

After menopause, vaginal dryness and reduced mucus production predispose women to vaginal, urethral, and urinary bladder infections. To treat whatever is causing the infection with antibiotics is only temporarily successful (and sometimes not at all successful) because the underlying and real cause of the problem is the inability of these parts of the body to resist infection, which is caused by a hormonal imbalance. For this reason, using a vaginal application of an estrogen cream works very well to restore hormone balance, with estriol being the most effective. A recent controlled trial of intravaginal estriol in postmenopausal women with recurrent urinary tract infections found that estriol significantly reduced the incidence of urinary infections compared to placebo (0.5 versus 5.9 episodes per year). In addition, estriol treatment resulted in the reemergence of friendly *Lactobacilli* bacteria and the near-elimination of colon bacteria, as well as the restoration of normal vaginal mucosa and a resumption of normal low pH (which inhibits the growth of many bacteria).

In my care of postmenopausal patients, there are those for whom estrogens are contraindicated by reason of a history of breast or uterine cancer and who are at risk of recurrent urinary tract and vaginal infections. I have been surprised to observe that those who opted for natural progesterone therapy have been remarkably free of these problems. Further, in many, their previous vaginal dryness and reduced mucus production returns to normal after three to four months of progesterone use. This suggests that natural progesterone also provides a direct benefit to vaginal and urethral tissues or may sensitize tissue receptors to the lowered levels of estrogens still present in postmenopausal women.

PELVIC INFLAMMATORY DISEASE (PID)

PID is a serious inflammation of the uterus and fallopian tubes that can result in pelvic abscesses, chronic pain, and infertility. Its treatment includes antibiotics for both sexual partners and, rarely, surgery. Some of the infections that can cause PID include gonorrhea, chlamydia, and coliform bacteria that come from the colon. The infection begins in the vagina and cervical tissues, then spreads up into the endometrium and out along the fallopian tubes, at which point the inflammation is called *salpingitis* or pelvic inflammatory disease (PID).

Preventing PID is dependent upon reducing the opportunity of vaginal contamination by wiping from front to back after a bowel movement, making sure sexual partners are uninfected, keeping the vaginal mucus healthy, and increasing your resistance to infections. In all of these tactics, vaginal mucus is an important factor. Normal vaginal mucus results from a normal balance of natural hormones and nutritional factors, such as vitamins beta-carotene, E, C, and B6, and the minerals zinc and magnesium. It is unlikely that synthetic hormones (contraceptive pills and menopausal hormones) provide the hormone balance or action necessary for the most balanced vaginal mucus.

Estriol is the estrogen most beneficial to vaginal and cervical tissue, the sites that act as the first line of defense against infection. Estriol is a product of estrone metabolism. Contraceptive synthetic estrogens, which inhibit the production of natural hormones, do not contain estriol and are not metabolized to form estriol. Progestins similarly inhibit production of natural progesterone.

After menopause, progesterone levels fall to near zero and estrone levels are also very low. Thus the protection against infection offered by estriol and progesterone is lost unless natural hormones are used in supplementation.

OVARIAN CYSTS AND *MITTELSCHMERZ*

Ovarian cysts are products of failed or disordered ovulation. As I have described earlier, one or more ovarian follicles is developed monthly by the effects of follicle-stimulating hormone (FSH). Luteinizing hormone (LH) promotes actual ovulation and the transformation of the follicle (after ovulation) into the corpus luteum, which produces progesterone. During a young woman's early years of menstruating, ovulation may coincide with a small amount of bleeding where the follicle has ruptured to release the egg. This can cause abdominal pain, often with a slight fever, at the time of ovulation (in the middle days between periods) and is commonly called *mittelschmerz* (German for "middle" and "pain"). Treatment might consist only of some ibuprofen, reassurance, rest, and perhaps a warm pack. It is unlikely to recur and portends no future problems.

Later in life, usually after their midthirties, women sometimes develop an ovarian cyst that may not cause any symptoms, or it may cause pelvic pain ranging from mild to severe. The cyst may simply collapse and disappear after a month or two, or it may persist and increase in size and discomfort during succeeding months. Such cysts are caused by a failed ovulation in which, for reasons presently unknown, the ovulation did not proceed to completion. With each succeeding month's surge of LH, the cyst swells and stretches the surface membrane, causing pain and possible bleeding at the site. Some cysts may become as large as a golf ball or lemon before discovery. Treatment may require surgery. (Removing the ovary along with the cyst used to be the standard procedure, but I recommend asking your surgeon to leave the ovary intact if at all possible.)

An alternative treatment for ovarian cysts is natural progesterone. The signaling mechanism that shuts off ovulation in one ovary each cycle is the production of progesterone in the other. If sufficient natural progesterone is supplemented prior to ovulation, LH levels are inhibited and both ovaries think the other one has ovulated, so regular ovulation does not occur. (This is the same effect as contraceptive pills.) Similarly, the high estriol and progesterone levels throughout pregnancy successfully inhibit ovarian activity for nine months. Therefore, adding natural progesterone from day 10 to day 26 of the cycle suppresses LH and its luteinizing effects. Thus the ovarian cyst will not be stimulated and, in the passage of one or two such monthly cycles, will very likely shrink and disappear without further treatment.

ENDOMETRIOSIS

Endometriosis is a serious condition in which tiny islets of endometrium (inner lining cells of the uterus) become scattered in areas where they don't belong: the fallopian tubes, within the uterine musculature (adenomyosis), and on the outer surface of the uterus and other pelvic organs, the colon, the bladder, and the sides of the pelvic cavity. With each monthly cycle, these islets of endometrium respond to ovarian hormones exactly as endometrial cells do within the uterus—they increase in size, swell with blood, and bleed into the surrounding tissue at menstruation. The bleeding (no matter how small) into the surrounding tissue causes inflammation and is very painful, often disabling. Symptoms begin seven to 12 days before menstruation and then become excruciatingly painful during menstruation. The pain may be diffuse and may cause painful intercourse or painful bowel movements, depending on the sites involved. Diagnosis is not easily established, as there is no lab test to identify endometrial islets, nor are they usually large enough to show on an X ray or sonogram. Laparoscopy (a minimally invasive surgery enabling a doctor to look into the abdomen with a small scope) is very useful in this regard.

The cause of endometriosis is unclear. Some authorities argue that these endometrial cells wander out through the fallopian tubes. Others suggest they are displaced through some sort of embryologic mix-up when an embryo is just forming its tissues. The fact is, however, that endometriosis seems to be a disease of the twentieth century. Given the severity of the pains and the association with monthly periods, it seems unlikely that earlier doctors would not have described the condition. Now that we know about xenoestrogens and the fact that the tissues of the developing embryo are especially sensitive to the toxic effects of xenoestrogens, it is tempting to speculate that our petrochemical age has spawned diseases we've never known before—and that endometriosis is one of them.

Mainstream treatment of endometriosis is difficult and not very successful. Surgical attempts at removing each and every endometrial implant throughout the pelvis is only temporarily successful. Many of the tiny islets are simply too small to see, and eventually they enlarge and the condition recurs. Another surgical venture is even more radical: the removal of both ovaries, the uterus and the fallopian tubes, the aim being to remove or reduce hormone levels as much as possible—not a pleasant prospect.

When women with endometriosis delay childbearing until their thirties, they are often unable to conceive. Pregnancy often retards the progress of the disease and occasionally cures it. With this in mind, other medical treatments attempt to create a state of pseudopregnancy, with long periods of supplemented progestins to simulate the high progesterone levels of pregnancy. Unfortunately, the high doses needed are often accompanied by side effects of the progestin and breakthrough bleeding.

As an alternative, I have treated a number of endometriosis patients, some after failed surgery, with natural progesterone and have observed considerable success. Since we know that estrogen initiates endometrial cell proliferation and the formation of blood vessel accumulation in the endometrium, the aim of treatment is to block this monthly estrogen stimulus to the aberrant endometrial islets. Progesterone stops further proliferation of endometrial cells. I advised such women to use natural progesterone cream from day six of the cycle to day 26 each month, using one ounce of the cream per week for three weeks, stopping just before their expected period. This treatment requires patience. Over time (four to six months), however, the monthly pains gradually subside as monthly bleeding in these islets becomes less and healing of the inflammatory sites occurs. The monthly discomfort may not disappear entirely but becomes more tolerable. Endometriosis is cured by menopause. This technique is surely worth giving a trial, since the alternatives are not all that successful and laden with undesirable consequences and side effects.

FIBROIDS

Otherwise known as *myoma* of the uterus, fibroids are the most common growth of the female genital tract. They are round, firm, benign (i.e., noncancerous) lumps of the muscular wall of the uterus, composed of smooth muscle and connective tissue, and are rarely solitary. Usually as small as a hen's egg, they commonly grow gradually to the size of an orange or grapefruit. The largest fibroid on record weighed over 100 pounds. They often cause or are coincidental with heavier periods, irregular bleeding, and/or painful periods. After menopause, they usually wither away.

Fibroids are also one of the most common reasons that women in their thirties and forties have a hysterectomy. Some particularly skillful surgeons are capable of removing only the fibroid, leaving the uterus intact, but they are the exception.

Here again, natural progesterone offers a better alternative. Fibroid tumors, like breast fibrocysts, are a product of estrogen dominance. Estrogen stimulates their growth, and lack of estrogen causes them to atrophy. Estrogen dominance is a much greater problem than recognized by contemporary medicine. Many women in their midthirties begin to have anovulatory (nonovulating) cycles. As they approach the decade before menopause, they are producing much less progesterone than expected, but still producing normal (or more) estrogen. They retain water and salt, their breasts swell and become fibrocystic, they gain weight (especially around the hips and torso), they become depressed and lose sex drive, their bones suffer mineral loss, and they develop fibroids. All are signs of estrogen dominance relative to a progesterone deficiency.

When sufficient natural progesterone is replaced, fibroid tumors no longer grow in size (they generally decrease in size) and can be kept from growing until menopause, after which they will atrophy. This is the effect of reversing estrogen dominance.

Anovulatory periods can be verified by checking serum or saliva progesterone levels the week following supposed ovulation. A low reading indicates lack of ovulation and the need to supplement with natural progesterone.

ENDOMETRIAL CANCER

This pelvic disorder is another example of estrogen dominance. Unopposed estrogen is the only known etiology of endometrial carcinoma. Both natural progesterone and the synthetic progestins give a protective effect from this disease. This important topic is discussed more thoroughly in Chapter 14, "Hormone Balance and Cancer."

EARLY MISCARRIAGES

Early miscarriages, also known as spontaneous abortions, are becoming more frequent. It is estimated that 25 percent of all pregnancies will miscarry, half of them before the eighth week. If a woman suffers three or more miscarriages in succession, the problem is termed "habitual" abortion. Only 15 percent of them can be traced to a specific maternal organic disease. The chief cause of early loss of pregnancy is now thought to be *luteal phase failure,* in which the ovarian production of progesterone fails to increase sufficiently during the first several weeks after fertilization. Maintaining the secretory endometrium (uterine lining) and the development of the embryo are dependent upon adequate luteal-supplied progesterone. The failure of progesterone production during this crucial time of pregnancy mirrors the rising incidence of progesterone deficiency occurring during ten or more years before menopause. While there may be a number of factors involved (such as stress or nutritional deficiencies), one such culprit may be exposure (even embryogenic) to xenoestrogens.

When a woman has experienced several early miscarriages and luteal phase failure is suspected, I have usually recommended progesterone supplementation (in addition to nutritional support) starting after ovulation (day 14 or so) and continued on (when pregnancy is confirmed by pregnancy blood tests) for two months. After two months, placenta-derived progesterone becomes dominant. Reducing the supplemental progesterone during the third month should be gradual so as to avoid any abrupt drop in progesterone levels. I have had some success with this approach, and I see no harm in trying it. Your doctor can easily monitor your progesterone levels with saliva hormone assays.

HYSTERECTOMY

I have included hysterectomy here because it almost always falls under the category of an iatrogenic (i.e., physician-induced) pelvic disorder. Total hysterectomy has come to mean the removal of a woman's uterus and ovaries. Technically, a hysterectomy is only the removal of the uterus and an *oophorectomy* or *ovariectomy* is the removal of the ovaries. Since women who have had hysterectomies go into instant, surgically induced menopause, they are immediately put on hormone replacement therapy.

Dr. Stanley West, chief of reproductive endocrinology and infertility at St. Vincent's Hospital in New York and the author of *The Hysterectomy Hoax,* believes that, in general, a hysterectomy is never necessary unless a woman has cancer. How did it come to be that every year 600,000 women are getting hysterectomies and over 500,000 of them are unnecessary? As West points out, it has more to do with outdated views of women than any physical problem women are having. West quotes an M.D. who gave a speech to the American College of Obstetrics and Gynecology in 1971 as saying, ". . . after the last planned pregnancy, the uterus becomes a useless, symptom-producing, potentially cancer-bearing organ and therefore should be removed." As recently as 1979, the head of the Harvard School of Public Health declared, "If a woman is thirty-five or forty years old and has an organ that is disease prone and of little or no further use, it might as well be removed." I'm sure these physicians have good intentions, or at least do not intend to harm their patients, but they are sadly misguided in using hysterectomy as a routine treatment.

Removal of the ovaries is also known in medical terminology as female castration. Think of how men would respond if their doctors wanted to remove their testicles and prostate gland once they had all the children they wanted, and then put them on synthetic testosterone drugs. It's almost inconceivable. And yet removing a woman's ovaries is no less a violation and has equally devastating consequences, not the least of which are the side effects of the synthetic hormones she is put on to replace her own. Removing the ovaries as a matter of course has gone somewhat out of fashion lately. Doctors now tell their patients that sparing the ovaries will allow them to keep producing hormones, but this is not accurate. The blood supply of the ovaries is a branch of the uterine artery that is ligated (cut and tied off) in the usual hysterectomy. The loss of this blood supply by the ovaries routinely results in loss of ovarian function. Even in cases in which the ovaries appear to be saved, they often quit functioning in two to three years. It is as if somehow the ovaries know there is no longer a uterus there and within a few years they atrophy and stop producing hormones. Hysterectomy means castration, whether or not the ovaries are involved.

Hysterectomy is lucrative for the physician doing the surgery, lucrative for the pharmaceutical companies supplying the replacement hormones (600,000 new lifelong customers each year!), and physically, mentally, and emotionally expensive for women who undergo them. The aftereffects of hysterectomy tend to be played down by the physicians who do them, but they are frequent and include fatigue, depression, headaches, heart palpitations, mood swings, hair loss, loss of sex drive, vaginal dryness, and urinary tract problems. Women who are put on estrogen after a hysterectomy have to cope with all the side effects of unopposed estrogen and, if a progestin is added, all those side effects as well.

Before you submit yourself to a hysterectomy, I strongly recommend you reconsider, unless you clearly have a malignant cancer. The leading reasons given for hysterectomies are fibroids, uterine prolapse (the uterus falls from its normal position), and endometriosis. As you have read here, fibroids and endometriosis can usually be effectively helped with some natural progesterone cream, and there are many other ways to deal with uterine prolapse. If you want all the details and reasons not to have a hysterectomy, read Dr. West's book, *The Hysterectomy Hoax*.

If you've already had a hysterectomy and are struggling with the side effects of synthetic hormone replacement therapy, ask your doctor to use natural hormones. I have my patients wean themselves off HRT by gradually (over a period of three to four months) reducing their dosage, while at the same time using progesterone cream. In those very few women who still have hot flashes or vaginal dryness, I give them some estrogen cream, usually estriol, to use intravaginally for a few months, and they are then able to taper that off.

STAYING NATURALLY HEALTHY

The monthly rise and fall of natural estrogen(s) and progesterone not only prepares your body for procreation, in the sense of ova production, but also predisposes you to be healthy. Many of women's pelvic complaints arise from an imbalance of their hormones. This imbalance is most often a deficiency of progesterone. There are many factors that bring this about: nutritional deficiencies, stress, environmental xenoestrogens, toxins, depletion of follicles, and the hormonal imbalance induced by contraceptive pills composed of synthetic hormones. Progesterone deficiency and estrogen dominance can be recognized and handily treated by supplementation of natural progesterone, especially when combined with diet and supplements.

Chapter 17

HORMONE BALANCE AND OTHER COMMON HEALTH PROBLEMS

Until rather recently, women's ailments were regarded simply as evidence of some design flaw or inherent weakness of women's constitution. Women who had ailments with causes unknown to their male doctors were often treated with a condescending pat on the hand and a prescription for a tranquilizer to calm fragile nerves. During my own time in medicine, a great change has occurred. In my medical school class (of 1955), there were 112 men and three women. Now women constitute 30 to 60 percent of medical school classes. The era of condescension and not-so-benign neglect is passing. Surely medical progress will soon catch up to the real causes of women's ailments.

We now know that hormone balance is an important factor in a woman's overall health. Estrogen, testosterone, and progesterone are potent substances. They affect every organ and tissue of the body. Their effects are both complementary and opposing to each other. The sum total of all their effects is dependent not only on the quantity of a given hormone, but also on the relative quantity or balance of the hormones in relation to each other. Understanding this will help us understand (and correct) conditions that we call women's ailments.

FIBROCYSTIC BREASTS

Many women present themselves to their doctors with breast swelling or tender, painful breasts occurring each month before their menstrual periods. Exam by palpation may find exquisitely tender lumps in the breast. Even though he knows with almost 100-percent certainty that the problem is due to fibrocystic breasts, the doctor is aware of the liability of overlooking any breast lump and therefore often orders a mammogram (especially painful in this condition). Mammogram readings are often couched in terms of caution and the advice to rule out potential underlying cancer. (Cancer lumps in breasts are rarely if ever painful.) A trial of vitamin E and avoiding caffeine and other methyl xanthines (coffee, tea, colas, chocolate) may have little or no result. Attempts at needle aspiration of the cyst are often bungled, sometimes causing painful bruising, and lead to a referral to a surgeon predisposed to surgery, who brings up the prospect of cancer and advises surgical removal of the offending cyst/tumor. If "merely" a cyst is found (and removed), the patient is supposed to feel grateful. She usually receives no other medical treatment for her cysts other than a suggestion to try warm packs and put up with her painful monthly exieriences.

If she makes the rounds of enough doctors, she will come across someone who wants her to take a drug (usually a testosterone analog) to suppress her excess estrogen. Besides being expensive, she finds that a few, mostly masculinizing side effects are part of the bargain: acne, seborrhea, hair growth on face and body, male pattern baldness, lower pitch to voice, vaginal dryness, and sagging, smaller breasts. Most women find the treatment is worse than the disease.

From my women patients, I learned that fibrocystic breasts were most often merely a sign of estrogen dominance; relatively high estrogen and low progesterone. In my experience, using natural progesterone routinely resolves the problem. I also recommend adding vitamin E in dosages of 600 IU at bedtime, supplemental magnesium (300 milligrams a day), and vitamin B6 (50 milligrams a day). I cannot recall a case in which the result was not positive. Once the cysts have cleared up, you can reduce the progesterone dose to find the smallest dose that is still effective each month and continue the treatment as needed through menopause. This treatment is simple, safe, inexpensive, successful, and natural.

MIGRAINE HEADACHES

Migraines are serious headaches, most often occurring only on one side of the head, which are often preceded by a vague sense (aura) that the sufferer learns to recognize as an impending headache. Migraines are thought to be related to overdilation of blood vessels in the brain. They very likely have an allergic or chemically mediated trigger and are related to stress. They vary in severity, sometimes becoming almost unendurable without narcotic medication, and can be accompanied by nausea and vomiting. Routine treatment involves ergotamine medication (often combined with caffeine), which, to achieve success, may result in side effects of muscle pains, numbness and tingling in the fingers and toes, rapid (or slowed) heart rate, and nausea and vomiting. Migraine victims live in fear of their next headache.

When migraine headaches occur with regularity in women only at premenstrual times, they are most likely due to estrogen dominance. These are the lucky patients. Estrogen causes dilation of blood vessels, and thus contributes to the cause(s) of migraines. One of the many virtues of natural progesterone is that it helps restore normal vascular tone, counteracting the blood vessel dilation that causes the headache. Here again, progesterone is safe and treats the cause in a normal, physiologic way. The more dangerous pharmaceutical drugs can be reserved for the rare case that does not respond completely to progesterone.

SKIN PROBLEMS (ACNE, SEBORRHEA, ROSACEA, PSORIASIS, AND KERATOSES)

Acne is more common in males than in females. It is especially common in males around and just after puberty. It may last for decades, but does not occur in eunuchs (castrated men). Androgens (testosterone and others) are involved in acne. Scattered throughout the skin, but more common around the hairline, nose, and ears, are little skin (sebaceous) follicles that make an oily wax known as *sebum*. Sebum keeps our skin smooth and supple. Extra androgens stimulate excess sebum production; drying sebum blocks the gland outlet at the skin surface, causing retention of sebum. A common benign bacterium (*Corynebacterium acnes*) multiplies in the incarcerated sebum, causing low-grade inflammation. Vitamin A deficiency can aggravate acne and make it more difficult to heal. Vitamin A or beta-carotene and zinc aid the resolution of acne. Many dermatologists prescribe tetracycline antibiotic because it inhibits bacterial growth and thus reduces inflammation. Tetracycline does not cure acne; it merely reduces the inflammation. It also kills friendly intestinal bacteria, leading to "leaky gut" syndrome and yeast overgrowth known as candida.

When a woman in her late thirties or early forties develops acne, I suspect increased androgen production. In almost all adult female patients with this condition, supplemental progesterone clears the skin. My hypothesis is that ovarian follicle depletion leading to progesterone deficiency results in increased adrenal production of androgens. When progesterone is resupplied, androgen production goes down and the skin clears. (The same hypothesis does not apply to men.) But in women, topical progesterone cream does wonders for acne.

Seborrhea is a related condition of the sebum-producing follicles. It causes flaking and itching skin without specific inflammation of the skin follicles. It, too, clears rapidly with topical progesterone cream.

Rosacea is a rose-colored, flaking inflammation of skin, usually on the face symmetrically adjacent to the nose or forehead, sometimes with itching. It tends to be chronic and recurring. Its cause is unknown, but I have seen it well controlled with vitamin B12 injections. Cortisone creams suppress the inflammation, but do not cure rosacea. Continued use of fluoridated cortisone preparations results in atrophy of skin cells with permanent detrimental results. My patients using topical progesterone who happened to have rosacea have applied the cream directly to affected skin areas and report excellent results, though I don't know what the mechanism of action could be.

Similarly, patients with psoriasis (a normally intractable skin disorder characterized by red, scaly patches) have reported impressive remissions of the condition when progesterone cream was applied. In some cases, psoriatic skin lesions that had been present for many years cleared completely. Since progesterone skin creams providing physiologic dosages have no side effects, I see no reason not to try it.

Keratoses are generally small skin lesions composed of dry, hardened skin cells (keratinized epithelial cells) in discrete patches or protuberances considered "hornlike" to early doctors. They are thought by some to be precursors of later squamous cell skin cancers. People spend considerable time and money having dermatologists remove them. My patients using progesterone cream report that keratoses soften and disappear when the cream is applied directly to them. (See Chapter 14, "Hormone Balance and Cancer," for details.)

HIGH BLOOD PRESSURE

Hypertension, or high blood pressure, undoubtedly has many causes. Estrogen dominance is one of them. Estrogen and progestins adversely affect cell membranes, resulting in sodium and water influx into cells (causing intracellular edema or water retention) and loss of potassium and magnesium. The net result is often hypertension. Dr. Milton G. Crane has extensively studied the effects of estrogen, progestins, and progesterone on cell membranes, plasma renin activity, high blood pressure, and aldosterone excretion rates. He has concluded that estrogen dominance and oral contraceptive agents are a major cause of hypertension in women.

This was borne out in my practice. The water retention caused by estrogen is the culprit. Since the extra water is contained within body cells and is not loose in the extracellular spaces, it is not effectively reduced by diuretics. In women not on contraceptive pills, estrogen dominance is synonymous with progesterone deficiency. When progesterone is resupplied, weight goes down (excess water is excreted) and blood pressure returns to normal. Patients report to me that after starting progesterone their diuretics suddenly started working. If you are on diuretics or other antihypertensive drugs and using progesterone, it is wise to monitor your blood pressure and reduce or eliminate your antihypertension drugs gradually as needed to prevent low blood pressure (hypotension).

CANDIDA

Candida, short for *Candida albicans,* refers to yeast that usually lives companionably on our skin and (sometimes) our mucous membranes. On mucous membranes (mucosa), candida form whitish patches visible to the eye. The patches do not scrape off easily and cause itching and irritation. In the mouths of babies and young children, candida infection is called *thrush.* Under normal conditions our immune system protects us very well from unwarranted yeast overgrowth. However, if our immune system is dysfunctional, candida overgrowth becomes rampant, infecting the mucous membranes of the intestinal tract, mouth, and lungs. Another factor in candida control is the many helpful bacteria that live with us. Bacteria and yeast compete for sustenance. Bacteria suppress candida growth. When these helpful bacteria are killed by prolonged, potent antibiotics, candida overgrowth can result.

Candida like to live in the vagina. They grow well wherever it is warm, moist, and well supplied with their favorite nutrient—glucose. Skin and vaginal mucus contain glucose. Estrogen dominance increases mucus glucose, thereby facilitating candida growth. In males, candida can survive (but not flourish) under the penis foreskin, sometimes causing an irritation and sometimes causing no discernible symptoms. In sexual intercourse, candida are easily passed from one partner to the other.

While numerous medications are very effective at suppressing candida growth, the conditions within the vagina are such that reinfection is probable. Candida are often found in the skin folds of the anus, from which they reinfect the vagina. Successful treatment of candida includes a diet low in sugar and simple carbohydrates, good hygiene and protection from reinfection by one's sexual partner by using condoms or douching after sex, appropriate treatment of one's self and sexual partners with an over-the-counter yeast infection remedy (ask your pharmacist), and correction of estrogen dominance in the woman. This correction is accomplished by supplemental natural progesterone. When hormone imbalance is restored to normal balance using progesterone, candida growth is less likely to persist. The normal benign bacteria are restored and the body heals itself of its candida population.

ALLERGIES

Potential allergy-causing substances are abundant in everyone's environment. They do not provoke an allergic response unless the allergen load exceeds our body's ability to deal with it. Adequate cortisone blocks the histamine response to allergens. Progesterone is the precursor not only to estrogen and testosterone, but also to all the corticosteroids made by the adrenal gland. Adrenal exhaustion is the result of stress, vitamin C deficiency, and progesterone deficiency. Many of my patients using progesterone tell me that their allergy problems are much reduced. One woman called me from her supermarket to tell me that when she walked by the aisle with all the decongestants and antihistamines, she suddenly realized that since she began using progesterone she had not been plagued by her chronic sinus congestion. This is not an isolated incident; it is a common experience of many patients.

ARTHRITIS

Athritis is a generic Greek word that usually means only that one's joints, or the tissue around one's joints, hurt or are inflamed. It does not refer to any specific cause or any specific mechanism of action. It is more a Greek translation of a symptom than a diagnosis.

If your joints ache, or the connective tissue around your joints aches, your doctor is inclined to call it arthritis and prescribe nonsteroidal anti-inflammatory drugs (NSAIDs) such as aspirin, ibuprofen, or any of a dozen similar medications. You must realize that your joint aching is not due to NSAID deficiency, and your doctor's prescription is merely treating symptoms, not causes.

Connective tissue aches and pains have a variety of causes. Some of them include:

- Nutritional deficiencies
- Repeated trauma to cartilage and the connective tissue that holds joints together (as in pianist's hands and fingers)
- Repeated strain causing microscopic tears in connective tissue around joints and tendon sheaths (like carpal tunnel syndrome)
- Inflammatory reactions to these connective tissue strains due to prostaglandin imbalance secondary to dietary choices (like too much milk and meat and not enough foods with omega-3 and omega-6 fatty acids)
- Lack of physiological cortisone responses to check the inflammatory reactions

This is where progesterone comes in. Natural progesterone has anti-inflammatory properties that the synthetic analogs do not have. Many, many of my patients using natural progesterone cream report relief of chronic aches and pains, and other doctors have also reported this to me. You can rub progesterone cream or oil directly on the joint or tissue that hurts. I do not have a good explanation for why it works, but the consistency of the reports makes me believe it does. Here is another excellent opportunity for research.

AUTOIMMUNE DISORDERS

Autoimmune disorders are those disease states in which your own antibodies attack some gland or tissue in your body. Normally your antibodies protect you from harmful invaders, but in this case they go after normal tissue. The actual cause is generally never found. Autoimmune disorders, in general, are more common in women. Why should this be? It is natural to suspect estrogen, the one hormone that is more plentiful in women than men over the course of a lifetime. After follicle depletion or menopause, some women make less progesterone than men of the same age. The onset of autoimmune disorders is often in middle age, when estrogen dominance becomes common. Hashimoto's thyroiditis, Sjögren's disease, Graves' disease (toxic goiter), and lupus erythematosus are all not only more common in women, but appear to be related to estrogen supplementation or estrogen dominance. Recent studies have shown that women who use hormone replacement therapy containing estrogen are more likely to get lupus.

Many of my patients with autoimmune disease who began using natural progesterone to relieve menopausal symptoms reported that their disease symptoms also gradually abated. This is a clinical question that haunts my mind: Is this an unrecognized symptom of estrogen toxicity, or the fact that progesterone itself may "tune down" the antibody-modulated disorder? Further research would be nice.

INFERTILITY

The use of natural progesterone can give women the power to enhance their fertility without a lot of expensive office visits and prescription hormones. It also flies in the face of mainstream medicine's approach to fertility, which doesn't trouble me since their success rate in achieving conception tends to be depressingly low. It's no wonder—they are prescribing the wrong hormones! Synthetic estrogens and progestins generally cause more problems than they solve.

I believe that estrogen dominance from progesterone deficiency has caused a near epidemic of infertility among women in their midthirties. Excess estrogen seems to stimulate the ovaries to overproduce follicles, which, combined with delayed childbearing, results in an early burnout of the follicles. If you are having difficulty conceiving, you may be able to use progesterone to your advantage.

I had a number of patients in my practice who had been unable to conceive. For two to four months I had them use natural progesterone from days five to 26 in the cycle (stopping on day 26 to bring on menstruation). Using the progesterone prior to ovulation effectively suppressed ovulation. After a few months of this, I had them stop progesterone use. If you still have follicles left, they seem to respond to a few months of suppression with enthusiasm, and the sucessful maturation and release of an egg. Some of my patients who had been been trying to conceive for years had very good luck conceiving with this method. There are even a few children named after me!

On the other side of this coin is the fact that using progesterone prior to ovulation can suppress ovulation. In a normal menstrual cycle, the release of progesterone by one ovary functions as a signal to the other ovary not to ovulate—Nature's brilliant plan for avoiding multiple births. If you're using progesterone cream prior to ovulation, chances are good both ovaries will interpret its presence as a sign that the other ovary has ovulated, thus effectively suppressing ovulation.

If you do decide to use progesterone while trying to conceive, be sure to begin using it only *after* you have ovulated each month. You can track your ovulation by taking your temperature each morning before you get out of bed. When you ovulate, the release of progesterone will cause a slight rise in body temperature. Once that has happened, you can safely continue using the progesterone cream.

If you think you may be pregnant and want the pregnancy, do *not* stop using the progesterone until you have done a pregnancy test, as a sudden drop in progesterone levels would signal the body to shed the uterine lining, possibly inducing an abortion. While the urine pregnancy tests you can buy at a drugstore are reliable after day 28 of your cycle, a blood pregnancy test is reliable within several days after conception. (You usually do not need a doctor's prescription to get a blood pregnancy test at a local medical lab.) If it is positive and you want to remain pregnant, you should continue to use progesterone cream to prevent the scheduled menstrual shedding and to protect the developing fetus from early miscarriage. Progesterone should be continued at least until the third month of pregnancy, when the placenta becomes the major producer of progesterone, at which time you can gradually taper your progesterone supplementation. If blood progesterone levels remain good, you can discontinue it altogether. By the third trimester, the placenta will be making hundreds of times more progesterone than you would be getting with the cream alone.

PART III

CREATING AND MAINTAINING HORMONE BALANCE

Chapter 18

HOW TO USE PROGESTERONE SUPPLEMENTATION

The purpose of this chapter is to review the types of progesterone available and to give you a specific guide for using progesterone. For the most part, how you use natural progesterone will depend first on whether you are premenopausal or menopausal rather than on your list of individual symptoms. If you're currently taking HRT or have migraines, you'll need more specific instructions, which are covered later in the chapter. The dosage you use and the exact days of your cycle (if you still have one) you use it will vary according to your individual biochemistry. I will review those criteria below.

As I've said elsewhere in the book, there are no known side effects of progesterone when it is taken in small physiological doses, that is, 20 to 40 milligrams per day. Very large doses can cause sleepiness, although most women report they simply feel calm. Enormous doses can cause an anesthetic or drunken effect. Some women report estrogen dominance symptoms for a week or two after starting progesterone, but this is caused by a sensitization of estrogen receptors and generally disappears within a few weeks. If you're still having periods and you take progesterone out of phase with your cycle, it may change the timing of your period or cause some spotting.

TYPES OF PROGESTERONE SUPPLEMENTATION

If progesterone supplementation is decided upon, a woman can choose between skin creams and oils, sublingual (i.e., under the tongue) drops, and capsules.

Creams and Oils

My preference among the various available forms of progesterone supplements remains the transdermal route, meaning "through the skin." My reasons have to do with the appropriateness of hormone supplementation. Remember that the goal is *physiologic* hormone *balance*. By physiologic, I mean that the dosages approximate (and not exceed) normal hormone needs and responses. When intervening in a system of biofeedback controls, it is unwise to exceed the normal responses of the healthy gland. In the case of hypothyroidism or adrenal deficiency, supplemental dosages greater than normal will suppress normal function of the target gland. Dr. William Jefferies, in his book *The Safe Uses of Cortisone,* makes this same point in a convincing manner. I try to follow the same principle in regard to estrogen and progesterone. In patients in whom I suspect progesterone deficiency, I choose dosages that approximate the ovaries' normal expected production of progesterone. What I am treating is progesterone deficiency secondary to follicle depletion. I do not wish to suppress whatever function of the ovary still remains.

The fact that transdermal progesterone is well absorbed, as

shown by the good concentration of it in target tissues such as breasts (see Chapter 14, "Hormone Balance and Cancer," and the section on breast cancer), without a demonstrable rise in plasma (blood) levels is perplexing to some. In fact, some doctors argue that because they give their patients progesterone cream, take a blood test a month later, and no rise in progesterone is shown, this is proof that progesterone is not well absorbed when applied on the skin. The explanation, however, is quite simple.

Progesterone is fat-soluble and, as such, is not soluble in the watery blood plasma, which is the part of the blood tested for hormone levels. Progesterone made in the ovaries is protein-bound, making it soluble in the plasma. However, protein-bound progesterone is only 1- to 9-percent biologically available. In contrast, when progesterone is absorbed across skin or mucous membranes (such as the mouth), it is not protein-bound and only a small fraction of it is found in plasma. The majority of it rides through the bloodstream on red blood cells, much as pollen is carried by bees, or seeds are carried by birds. There it is nicely compatible with cholesterol, vitamin A, vitamin E, and other components of the fatty structure of the cell membrane. Furthermore, progesterone carried in this manner is close to 100-percent biologically available, as shown by salivary hormone assays.

Transdermal progesterone is absorbed through the skin into the underlying fat layer, from which it diffuses into the capillaries permeating the fat, where it can be taken up in the blood as needed. Further, the beneficial skin-moisturizing effects of transdermal progesterone are often much appreciated by the women using it.

Transdermal progesterone comes in creams and oils. The oils can be thick and sticky used transdermally; you can dilute them with olive oil at the time you are using them, or simply rub the oil briskly into your palms, where it is quickly absorbed.

Transdermal progesterone cream is very easily and quickly absorbed into the body, so you can apply it almost anywhere with success. However, I do recommend rotating the areas you apply it to avoid saturating any one area. It is best absorbed where the skin is relatively thin and well supplied with capillary blood flow, such as the face, neck, upper chest, breasts, inner arms and thighs, and the palms of the hands and soles of the feet.

Sublingual or Buccal Drops or Oil

Progesterone comes in a vitamin E oil that can be put in the mouth and held there (without swallowing) for a few minutes. It is important not to swallow for at least a minute after applying the drops this way so the drops are absorbed rather than swallowed. If not swallowed, they are absorbed through the mucous membranes of your mouth within minutes, leading to prompt elevation of progesterone levels. However, the levels fall in three to four hours due to rapid metabolizing and excretion, or absorption by body fat. Thus, to maintain a stable blood levels, the drops should be administered three to four times a day. The number of drops to be applied varies with the product, so you'll need to follow the directions on the label and experiment to find out what works best for you.

These types of liquid oil formulations can also be applied to the skin.

Capsules

The disadvantage of taking oral (by mouth) capsules is that they need to be given in very large doses, 100 to 200 milligrams per day, to compensate for the 85 to 90 percent that will be excreted almost immediately through the liver. This is 10 to 20 times greater than transdermal doses just to get the 20 to 24 milligrams needed daily. I see no reason to put the liver to all this work just to get 10 to 15 percent of the progesterone into the bloodstream.

When progesterone is taken orally, it (like other fat-soluble nutrients) is taken up by the portal vein, which transports it directly to the liver, where much of it is metabolized and conjugated (combined with glucuronide) for excretion in bile. This is termed the "first pass loss" through the liver. Some undoubtedly is absorbed by chylomicrons, tiny bits of fat that float in the bloodstream, and will circulate through the body, but the rate at which this happens varies greatly according to the health of the digestive tract and liver, stress levels, diet, and many other factors, including basic individual biochemistry, and thus it is unpredictable. In general, oral doses of progesterone (even in the micronized versions) must be greater than transdermal doses to create the equivalent biologic effects. For example, the success of Dr. Joel Hargrove from Vanderbilt University in using progesterone for PMS requires 300 to 400 milligrams or more per day to accomplish what I have observed in patients using only 30 to 40 milligrams per day by the transdermal route.

Because of the great safety of progesterone and the freedom from side effects, I am not aware of any danger in using the larger oral dosages. However, I see no reason to subject the liver to this extra work. In addition, I have had women taking oral progesterone complain that it makes them sleepy, indicating that they are getting a larger dose than needed. I have a further concern that liver-generated metabolites of oral progesterone may have diminished or different effects from the natural progesterone molecule.

TESTING YOUR HORMONE LEVELS

Saliva Testing

The usual way to test hormone levels has been with a blood test that measures the blood serum or blood plasma content of the hormones. These tests have been somewhat unreliable because they do not give your biologically active hormone levels, and progesterone creams can take weeks to show up in serum in spite of the fact that they begin having an effect within hours of being used.

Hormones made in the ovaries, testes, or adrenals are wrapped in protein envelopes called either sex hormone–binding globulin (SHBG) or cortisol-binding globulin (CBG) so they can be carried in the blood. These protein-bound hormones are not fully biologically active. The more important and relevant hormone levels are the 1 to 10 percent that are unbound and thus biologically active. Saliva contains only the unbound, biologically active hormone molecules. When progesterone is absorbed through the skin, it is not coated with protein and is carried in the blood's fatty components, such as chylomicrons or red blood cell membranes. Thus, even though progesterone from skin creams is slow to appear in the serum, it is found to be quickly present (within hours) in saliva, indicating that it is well absorbed and available to cells in biologically active form.

Saliva testing is quicker, less expensive, and less painful than blood tests, and is a reliable way for your doctor to measure hormone levels and test for hormone deficiencies. It will confirm that the hormones you are taking are being absorbed and utilized; it doesn't involve a trip to a lab or drawing blood; and it's inexpensive enough that you can do a number of tests, such as over the course of a day or a month. For those women who wish to monitor their own hormone levels to find out if they are ovulating, for example, the tests can be ordered and easily done at home without a doctor's prescription.

Salivary testing done by Dr. David Zava at Aeron Lab to test the absorption of transdermal progesterone creams confirms my hunch that this form works better than other methods or routes because the hormone is absorbed more efficiently, the effect is longer-lasting, and it doesn't create the highs and lows created with the oral (swallowed) or sublingual (held in the mouth) drops. While these latter two forms are absorbed even faster than the creams, they are also excreted faster. My guess is that the interrupted highs and lows of a hormone like progesterone is confusing to the hypothalamus, leading to physiologic levels that may actually "tune down" or down regulate the receptor response. My goal is to be able to mimic normal physiologic levels of progesterone, to simulate what the ovaries would be doing if their follicles were in working order.

For a list of labs that do salivary testing of hormones, turn to the Resources section on page 334.

Blood Serum or Plasma Testing

Serum levels of progesterone will rise in about three months of proper use of progesterone cream. If your doctor wants to measure your serum progesterone levels, here are some guidelines: Normal, untreated (not on HRT) postmenopausal patients will show an initial serum progesterone level of 0.03 to 0.3 ng/ml, and after three months of transdermal progesterone, this level rises to 3 to 4 ng/ml, or about 10 times higher. In normal premenopausal women, luteal (midcycle) phase progesterone levels are 7 to 28 ng/ml, a level usually sufficient to sustain the specialized lining in the uterus prepared each month to receive the fertilized egg and nourish the developing embryo. In treating osteoporosis, for example, it is not necessary to reach these levels. Good results are obtained at progesterone levels of 3 to 4 ng/ml.

NOT ALL "WILD YAM EXTRACT" IS PROGESTERONE

One word of caution: Not all products with labels claiming

"wild yam extract" actually contain any progesterone. By historical practice, many nutritional products have merely listed their ingredients by such nonspecific labeling. Progesterone is obtained by extracting specific components from plants (e.g., diosgenin from wild yams or soybeans) and then converting them to actual progesterone in the laboratory. As I mentioned in earlier chapters, the synthetic progestins are also made from diosgenin. The key difference is that their molecular structure is not found in nature, and certainly not in the female body!

Progesterone (U.S. Pharmacopeia) is available on the wholesale pharmaceutical market. It is used by the major pharmaceutical companies as the base from which they synthesize their estrogen, testosterone, cortisone, and, of course, their progestin products. Unfortunately, the early alternative nutritional companies who incorporated this same progesterone in their products saw fit to list it as "extract of wild yam." Now, with the success of progesterone supplementation, many companies are producing products listed as containing wild yam extract, but they actually contain no progesterone. What many of these "wild yam extract" products contain is diosgenin, which is indeed the *laboratory* precursor to progesterone and other hormones, but there is no evidence that the human body converts diosgenin to hormones. In fact, rodent and human studies of diosgenin supplementation only show that it sometimes creates a drop in cholesterol levels. It may very well be that the human body converts some of the diosgenin to hormones or has phytoestrogenic or progestogenic action, but this action would be unpredictable and vary widely from person to person.

Another word of caution: Even when a cream contains progesterone, it will not be effective if it isn't suspended in the proper medium. Products containing mineral oil will prevent the progesterone from being absorbed into the skin. Other products haven't properly stabilized the progesterone, so it deteriorates over time with exposure to oxygen, and by the time you get to the bottom of the jar, you aren't getting any progesterone. (Some natural progesterone creams are sold in a tube instead of a jar, reducing their exposure to oxygen and thus possibly ensuring that they retain more potency over time.) The table below is an independent laboratory assay of products claiming to contain progesterone or "wild yam extract." Amounts below 800 milligrams per two-ounce jar will not supply sufficient progesterone if you are truly deficient. My advice is to purchase your progesterone cream accordingly!

RANGE OF PROGESTERONE CONTENT
OF BODY CREAMS & OILS
(IN ALPHABETICAL ORDER)

I. Creams/Oils Containing 2000 to 3000 mg Progesterone per Ounce

Progest-E Complex	Ray Peat	Eugene, OR

II. Creams/Oils Containing More than 400 mg Progesterone per Ounce (800 mg per two-ounce jar or tube)

Bio Balance	Elan Vitale	Scottsdale, AZ
Happy PMS	HM Enterprises, Inc.	Norcross, CA
NatraGest	Broadmore Labs, Inc.	Ventura, CA
PhytoGest	Karuna Corporation	Novato, CA
Pro-Alo	HealthWatchers Systems	Scottsdale, AZ
Pro-Gest	Professional & Technical Services, Inc.	Portland, OR

III. Creams/Oils Containing 2 to 15 mg Progesterone per Ounce

Life Changes	MW Labs	Atlanta, GA
Endocreme	Wuliton Labs	Palmyra, MO
Pro-Dermex	Gero Vita International	Reno, NV

IV. Creams Containing Less than 2 mg Progesterone per One Ounce

Born Again	Phytopharmica	Green Bay, WI
Femarone	Wise Essen. Inc.	Minneapolis, MN
Menopause Form	PMS Relief, Inc.	Auburn, CA
Nutri-Gest	NutriSupplies	West Palm Beach, FL
PMS Formula	PMS Relief, Inc.	Auburn, CA
Progestone-HP	Dixie Health, Inc.	Atlanta, GA
Progerone	Nature's Nutrition, Inc.	Vero Beach, FL
Wild Yam Cream	Alvin Last, Inc.	Yonkers, NY
Yamcon	Phillips Nutritionals	Laguna Hills, CA

An independent laboratory assay prepared by Aeron Lifecycles, San Leandro, CA, 7/31/95.

WHEN TO USE NATURAL PROGESTERONE

As I've mentioned throughout the book, in Western industrialized cultures, pharmaceutical companies buy natural progesterone (derived from yams or soybeans), and then chemically alter its molecular form to produce the various progestins, which, *not* being found in nature, are patentable and therefore more profitable. Most physicians are unaware that their prescription progestins are made from progesterone (from yams or soybeans) and that natural progesterone is available, safer than progestins, more effective, and relatively inexpensive.

Whether or not to use natural progesterone when a woman is premenopausal is a decision best made by each individual woman working with a health care professional familiar with female hormones and the use of natural progesterone, and based on the signs and symptoms of estrogen dominance that follows.

Signs and Symptoms of Estrogen Dominance in a Premenopausal Woman

- Water retention, edema (swelling, bloating)
- Fatigue, lack of energy
- Breast swelling, fibrocystic breasts
- Premenstrual mood swings, depression
- Loss of sex drive
- Heavy or irregular menses
- Uterine fibroids
- Craving for sweets
- Weight gain, fat deposition at hips and thighs
- Symptoms of low thyroid such as cold hands and feet

HOW MUCH NATURAL PROGESTERONE TO USE

Depending upon the amount of progesterone in the jar or tube, you'll want to use anywhere from 1/8 to 1/2 teaspoon of the cream per day, or three to 10 drops of the oil.

Normal production of progesterone during the middle of a normal menstrual cycle is 20 to 24 milligrams a day for 12 to 14 days. Thus, normal progesterone production during a menstrual month is 250 milligrams or so.

Let's say each two-ounce jar or tube of 3 percent (by volume) or 1.6 percent (by weight) progesterone cream contains 950 milligrams. Thus one-half of a two-ounce jar or tube would be more than sufficient to maintain adequate progesterone needs in a postmenopausal woman for one month. This would amount to 20 to 30 milligrams per day.

The best way to tell if enough is being used is whether your symptoms are relieved. For example, when estrogen dominance exists throughout the menstrual month, water retention and weight gain occur in the week before menstruation. After sufficient progesterone is supplemented, this cyclic weight gain no longer occurs. If you are menopausal and experiencing hot flashes or vaginal dryness, you will certainly know if those symptoms improve.

Since there are varying amounts of progesterone in the creams, and every woman's biochemistry and ability to absorb and use the cream are different, the actual dose will vary. Since natural progesterone is notable for its freedom from side effects, such latitude in dosing carries no risk.

For premenopausal women, stopping the cream at day 26 or 28 usually results in a normal menstrual period within 48 hours or so.

For menopausal women, a short period of not using the hormone tends to maintain receptor sensitivity. Since many postmenopausal patients do not begin supplementation until after a number of years of deficiency, and since much of this fat-soluble hormone will be initially "lost" in body fat, it is wise to use the full two-ounce monthly dose for three months or so to overcome the deficiency state. After this, dosage can usually be reduced.

The cream can be applied to the palms of the hands, the face and neck, the upper chest and breast, the inside of the arms, and behind the knees. Rotating among the various sites will maximize absorption. The size of the "gob" to use will become apparent as one proceeds through each monthly cycle.

Premenopausal women can use progesterone approximately two weeks per month. Since normal progesterone production can reach 20 milligrams per day between days 15 to 26 of the cycle (day one being the onset of bleeding), I usually begin by recommending the cream be used between day 12 and day 26 to approximate normal levels. Some women whose cycles are naturally longer will use it from day 10 to day 28.

Some doctors will prescribe estrogen for premenopausal women with irregular bleeding. However, there is no reason to give estrogen of any sort to a woman who is still having menstrual bleeding. The fact of menstrual bleeding means there is no estrogen deficiency. Menstrual periods may be irregular due to progesterone deficiency. If you have been put on estrogen for irregular periods, taper down the estrogen and start using progesterone cream as described above.

If bleeding starts before day 26 (or before it would normally begin), stop the progesterone and start counting up to day 12 again, and then start the progesterone again. It may take three cycles before you achieve synchrony with your normal cycle.

Menopausal women not receiving estrogen supplementation have an even wider latitude in using progesterone cream. For convenience, they may choose to select a dosage schedule based on the calendar month. The cream may be applied over a 14- to 21-day time period and then discontinued until the next month.

Menopausal women taking a cyclic estrogen supplement should reduce their dosage to one-half when starting the progesterone. Since progesterone replacement in women deficient in progesterone may initially (and temporarily) increase the sensitivity of estrogen receptors, it's important to reduce the dosage by one-half immediately. If you do not, you are likely to experience symptoms of estrogen dominance during the first one to two months of progesterone use.

An abrupt reduction in estrogen can trigger resumption of hot flashes or vaginal dryness. These symptoms can be prevented by gradual lowering of the dose. There are several ways to reduce your dose of estrogen. I usually recommend reducing the dose by one-half when starting the progesterone. Then every two to three months you can try lowering the dose by half again. If the estrogen pill can be broken in half, the process is simple. If the estrogen pill is not easily broken in half (such as Premarin), you can take one every other day, every third day, and so forth.

Estrogen and progesterone can be used together during a three-week or 24- to 25-day time period each month, leaving five to seven days each month without either hormone. The estrogen dose should be low enough that monthly bleeding does not occur but high enough to prevent vaginal dryness or hot flashes.

As I discussed above, hot flashes are not a sign of estrogen deficiency per se. They are a sign of lack of estrogen and/or progesterone response to the urgings of hypothalamic centers (the GnRH prompt). Often when progesterone levels are raised, the pituitary stops trying to signal the ovaries to ovulate, the hypothalamus settles down, and the hot flashes usually subside.

(Note: If your physician wants to test the validity of this mechanism, the FSH and LH levels before and after adequate progesterone supplementation can be measured. A decline in FSH and LH indicates that the GnRH prompt has subsided.)

I recommend you have a goal of getting off estrogen altogether. You can experiment with lowering the estrogen dose until you find the lowest dose that prevents vaginal dryness (my preference is a vaginal cream of estriol) and/or hot flashes. Since postmenopausal women continue to make estrogen (primarily in their body fat), many women find that estrogen supplementation can be eliminated altogether five to six months after starting the progesterone. The presence of progesterone makes estrogen receptors more sensitive, so that your own (endogenous) estrogen is sufficient. In this process of lowering your estrogen dose, you may have to ask your doctor to prescribe smaller doses of pills or capsules, since some are difficult or impossible to break into halves or quarters.

If you are using Estraderm patches, you should be aware they come in two dosages. Generally, both dosages are too high; my patients experienced breast fullness and tenderness and water retention even when using the lower-dose patch. Physicians familiar with alternative health care approaches have access to compounding pharmacies which can make a natural estrogen cream, which is another approach.

Menopausal women taking an estrogen and progestin combination should stop the progestin immediately when progesterone cream is added. For example, if you are taking Premarin and Provera, the most common combination, you should stop taking the Provera. I have found no ill effects in stopping Provera abruptly.

Again, the estrogen should be tapered slowly. There are now some estrogen/progestins combined in one pill, but I don't recommend these as it's important to go off the progestin when you start using progesterone cream.

USING PROGESTERONE IF YOU HAVE MIGRAINES

As mentioned earlier, when migraine headaches occur premenstrually in women, they are often caused by estrogen dominance. Estrogen causes dilation of blood vessels, and thus contributes to the cause(s) of migraines. Natural progesterone helps restore normal vascular tone, counteracting the blood vessel dilation that causes the headache. If you have premenstrual migraines, try using progesterone during the ten days before your period. Be alert to the aura that usually precedes these headaches. If one occurs, you can apply a small glob (1/4 to 1/2 teaspoon) every three to four hours until your symptoms subside. This commonly requires only one or two extra applications. Higher doses of progesterone can be reached quickly with sublingual drops (progesterone in vitamin E oil), which are more rapidly absorbed (within minutes) than skin cream (usually within an hour or so), and thus may be more effective.

IF I'M MENOPAUSAL AND TAKE PROGESTERONE, WILL MY PERIODS START AGAIN?

Not usually. The buildup of blood in the uterus is strictly a function of estrogen. At menopause, your production of estrogen does not fall to zero; it falls to a level just below that needed for monthly periods. It is likely, however, that your progesterone production is very close to zero. Without progesterone, estrogen receptors are less sensitive. When progesterone is resumed, estrogen receptors become more sensitive, that is, more likely to respond to estrogen. Thus some women may notice that after a week or two of progesterone some vaginal bleeding may occur due to their own estrogen. At that point, a woman may stop the progesterone for a week and then start up again for three weeks, as she would if she were still menstruating. The cycle should be three weeks on progesterone and one week off. During the week off progesterone, there may be some bleeding. This is due to the persistence of estrogen production, which will diminish over time. This is the advantage of stopping progesterone for one week each month: It allows the estrogen-induced blood buildup to be shed.

Later, when no monthly bleeding occurs, the progesterone can be continued on a calendar basis: 24 days of progesterone and then stopping for the remainder of the month.

In cases of persistent spotting or vaginal bleeding (more than three months), consult your physician.

Chapter 19

THE HORMONE BALANCE PROGRAM

Most of the rest of the book has been devoted to explaining *why* your hormones are out of balance. This chapter will tell you how to bring your hormones back into balance. As I mentioned in the introduction to this book, I don't want you to think of progesterone as a magic bullet or a magic pill. Just taking the simple steps in this chapter to change your diet and lifestyle may very well be enough to bring your hormones back into balance. When we provide an optimum environment, our bodies are remarkably resilient and capable of healing themselves and restoring balance.

Menopause and premenopause are not diseases. They are natural biological processes that have gone awry in some women because of a less-than-optimum environment. My goal in this chapter is to show you how to create the healthiest possible environment for yourself. And I want you to know that, regardless of what your lifestyle has been in the past, it is *never* too late to get healthier. Every small step you take toward improving your health will make a big difference.

If you've spent decades eating refined and processed foods, avoiding exercise, and being exposed to xenoestrogens, taking these steps toward hormone balance may seem challenging at first. Changing habits is not always easy, and many of the processed foods are comfort foods we eat when we're upset or need to nurture ourselves. This holds especially true for chips, candy, cookies, ice cream, and baked goods. If you know what your comfort foods are, please don't try to eliminate them suddenly and completely from your diet. That's too harsh a step for most of us. If we are eating certain foods to nurture ourselves, then suddenly yank them away, all those parts inside we're trying to nurture are going to rebel. And you know what that means— obsessing about the food, bingeing, and guilt. That's as unhealthy as just continuing to eat the food.

Instead, gradually cut down on the amount you eat. Eat two cookies instead of ten. Eat one-fourth of a bag of chips instead of the whole bag. Eat a Hershey's kiss instead of a Hershey's bar. Begin to think of these foods as occasional treats rather than daily sustenance while you find other ways to nurture yourself. As your hormones begin to come back into balance and your blood sugar begins to stabilize, you'll find you have much less craving for sweet and salty junk food.

Do I need to tell anyone, again, that they should quit smoking? Just in case, if you're smoking, quit. Now.

I have nothing against alcohol consumption, but I recommend you limit it to no more than a two drinks a day. More than that will take a toll on your liver, deplete you of nutrients, and put you at a higher risk for cancer.

AVOID HYDROGENATED OILS AND MOST VEGETABLE OILS

Much of our fat has been processed into oils that differ greatly from the natural oils from which they are derived. The processing of these oils uses heat, high-pressure pressing, degumming (removing lecithin, complex carbohydrates, chlorophyll, calcium, magnesium, iron, and copper), alkylization (removing free fatty acids), bleaching (losing beta-carotene and chlorophyll), deodorizing (eliminating vitamin E and adding synthetic antioxidants and defoamers), and often hydrogenation (transforming oils into solid or semisolid masses of fats never found in nature). The altered fats and oils so produced are synthetic and foreign to nature. The term for natural fats and oils is *cis*-fatty acids, and the term for the unnatural, altered form of fats and oils is *trans*fatty acids. The foreign nature of the molecules of processed fats and oils correlates into deleterious effects on cell membranes and immune function, and other toxic effects, including cancer. Transfatty acids = higher cancer and heart disease risk. Most transfatty acids are listed on labels as hydrogenated or partially hydrogenated oils, and they are found in nearly all processed foods.

One of the single most important steps you can take toward better health is to eliminate refined oils from your diet as much as possible. This means hydrogenated oils, partially hydrogenated oils, and refined vegetable oils such as safflower and corn oil. Yes, this means staying away from margarine. I realize you have been told for many decades now that these oils are better for you than butter or lard, but this is marketing and advertising hype that is not based on science or truth. The hydrogenated oils found in margarine, potato chips, baked goods, candies, and other processed foods have as strong or stronger a link to heart disease as the animal fats and other saturated fats. The transfatty acids found in these oils actually damage the arteries.

The unsaturated vegetable oils that come in a clear bottle contain a double whammy: They are nearly always rancid, and the refining process has depleted them of their nutrients. The unsaturated vegetable oils (e.g., corn and safflower) and most of the nut and seed oils (e.g., sunflower and peanut) are so unstable that they are probably already rancid by the time you open the bottle, and are definitely rancid within hours of opening the bottle. Rancid oil is notorious for creating oxidation in the body, a chain reaction similar to rusting metal or the brown color that forms on a cut-up apple. These kinds of oxidative reactions are thought to be partially responsible for much of our chronic illness, including heart disease and cancer. The negative effects of oxidation are why antioxidant vitamins have become so popular.

Removing the nutrients from vegetable oils also removes their benefits. When they're fresh and unrefined, they contain all kinds of important vitamins and minerals, including vitamin E. Some vegetable oils are preserved with vitamin E, which is better than unpreserved, but I'd still prefer you avoid them altogether. (It is ironic that our foods, which in their fresh, whole state naturally contain preservatives such as vitamins C and E, are stripped of nutrients when they are processed, and then synthetic preservatives such as BHT are added back in.)

WHICH FATS AND OILS SHOULD YOU EAT?

There are, of course, "good" fats and oils. A few are essential, in the sense that our bodies need them and cannot make them from other foods we eat. These can be obtained in sufficient quantity by eating plenty of fresh vegetables and whole grains. Fish is also a good source of essential fats.

Olive oil also has a long history of being healthy. A study published in the *Journal of the National Cancer Institute* reports that olive oil lowers the risk of breast cancer. Dr. Dimitrios Trichopoulos of the Harvard School of Public Health, a coordinator of that study, cautions that the lesson of the study is not that we should add olive oil to what we normally eat, but that we should substitute olive oil for other fats and oils in our diet. In addition, the study found that women who ate the most vegetables and fruit had 48 percent less breast cancer compared to the group that ate the least. If a drug was shown to be that protective, every woman in North America and Europe would run out and buy it!

Try to eat the majority of your fats and oils as olive oil or butter. I know it is near heresy to recommend butter, but butter is only bad if you eat it in excess. A little butter on your toast in the morning is going to satisfy your craving for fats and is not going to hurt you because it's a stable, saturated fat. Saturated fat per se is *not* bad for you. It is an *excess* of saturated fat that is bad for you. When you eat more fat than you can burn off, you become fat and you create other imbalances in your body, including hormone imbalances. Don't blame the butter; blame the excess intake. If you can keep your fat calories to about 20 to 25 percent of your total calories, you won't have to worry about saturated fat (although it is preferable to keep red meat consumption to a minimum, which I'll explain shortly).

Olive oil is a monounsaturated fat, so it is stable and not subject to oxidation reactions. Please buy the green olive oil (usually the extra virgin), which is unrefined and still has all or most of its nutrients. Recent studies have shown that certain Greek and Italian populations with a very low incidence of heart disease have a high percentage of fat in their diet, but most of it is olive oil. The important thing to remember is that the Greeks and Italians are eating *unrefined* olive oil. Please follow suit. Your health is worth the extra money.

If you want to use oils in baking, use olive oil, butter, or coconut oil. Contrary to popular opinion, *unrefined* coconut oil (as opposed to the highly processed form most often used in prepared foods) is not at all bad for you, any more than butter is. In fact, equatorial people whose main source of fat is unrefined coconut oil tend to be very free of heart disease. Coconut oil is a very stable saturated oil that is excellent for cooking. But again, look for a white, unrefined coconut oil (it should not be yellow in color). Omega and Spectrum are two companies that sell unrefined coconut oil that you can find or order at most health food stores.

Canola oil is also a monounsaturated fat like olive oil, so it is stable but highly refined. It comes from the rapeseed plant and used to be called rapeseed oil, but the name didn't encourage consumer interest so it was changed to canola oil. Before canola oil can be sold for human consumption, a toxic ingredient in it needs to be removed. If you need a light, mild oil for baking, canola oil may be your best choice, but please don't make it a steady part of your diet. If you have a yen for chips, look for those made with canola oil.

EAT WHOLE, UNPROCESSED FOODS

If I had to choose one single piece of advice to give you that would most improve your health (assuming you are already a nonsmoker), it would be to learn to eat fresh, whole, unprocessed foods. They contain all the vitamins, minerals, and other nutrients you need, in abundance. They contain fiber, which is very important for hormone balance. And they don't contain refined white flour or sugar, additives, perservatives, or coloring.

When you were a kid, did you ever make glue out of white flour and water? Glue is what refined grains (wheat, rice, and corn, primarily) behave like in your digestive system. Most of the nutrients are stripped from them, and they gum up your digestive tract, interfering with the absorption of nutrients and giving you constipation.

What does eating whole foods mean? It means eating whole grains such as brown rice, bulgur, millet, quinoa, and amaranth (really a seed), which are tasty and can be used by themselves or in casseroles. It means eating whole grain (not just whole wheat) breads. It means eating beans, especially including soybean products. Beans do not need to cause gas if you introduce them gradually into your diet, soak them overnight, and discard the soaking water before cooking. They only take an hour or so to cook, if you soak them first. You can also use a product called Beano, which contains the enzyme necessary to digest beans, until your own body learns to make the enzymes. Most health food stores carry Beano. The phytoestrogens in soy products such as soy milk, miso, tofu, and tempeh are known to inhibit the growth of cancer. The Japanese, whose diet is very high in soy, tend to have very low rates of breast and prostate cancer.

Eating whole, unprocessed foods means emphasizing fresh vegetables. The awful habit of boiling vegetables until they're mushy and tasteless has given them a bad name. Fresh vegetables are delicious raw or lightly steamed. Fresh root vegetables, such as beets, carrots, turnips, onions, garlic, and potatoes, are wonderful baked with some olive oil and fresh herbs. Experiment with some of the more exotic green leafy vegetables, such as kale and bok choy. Once you become acquainted with these foods, you will find they are quick and simple to prepare, and very tasty.

And last but not least, eating whole, unprocessed foods means eating fresh fruit instead of desserts with white sugar—or with fructose, corn syrup, brown sugar, maple syrup, or honey. Sorry, but it's still all sugar. Before you balk at the idea of spending money on some expensive grapes or a papaya, stop and think how much you would pay for a pie, cake, or ice cream. If you really have a sweet tooth, try sprinkling apples, pears, or peaches with cinnamon, and baking them. Even then, your consumption of fruits shouldn't be overdone. They are primarily sugar, which will be turned into fat in your body if you don't burn it off.

If your diet is primarily refined and processed foods, make the change to whole foods gradually. Your digestive system needs time to adjust to the incease in fiber, and you need time to adjust to a new lifetsyle.

EAT ORGANIC FOODS WHENEVER POSSIBLE

If you're eating whole foods, emphasizing plenty of whole grains, fresh fruit, and vegetables, you'll be getting most of the nutrients you need—especially if the food is organic. Many nonorganic foods are grown in depleted soils without the minerals you need and are stored for long periods of time, which additionally depletes their vitamin content. Depleted soils grow weak, disease-prone plants that then get sprayed with pesticides.

Organic foods, on the other hand, need to be grown in good soil so they can more naturally resist predators and disease. They tend to be locally grown, and fresh. If you have a farmers' market in your area, take full advantage of it. You can usually find plenty of organic foods at reasonable prices because you're buying them directly from the grower. If you don't have a farmer's market, start one! Or tell the produce manager at your local supermarket that you would like organic produce. There are health food supermarkets springing up all around the country that feature hormone-free meat, whole foods, and organic produce. If there's one in your area, it will be worth the extra few dollars a week to shop there. Think of it as a long-term investment in your health.

ARE YOU ALLERGIC TO DAIRY PRODUCTS?

The promotion of milk as a healthy food is another example of the triumph of advertising and marketing over science and truth. New studies are showing that cows' milk may be responsible for a good deal of the juvenile diabetes in Western cultures, something alternative health care practitioners have been saying for decades. The current theory is that certain proteins in cows' milk set off an autoimmune reaction in the pancreas that eventually destroys that organ's ability to make insulin. Most children are allergic to cows' milk. They won't necessarily show their allergies by breaking out in hives—allergies can manifest in many other ways. I suspect that the incidence of childhood ear infections, diarrhea, and chronic sinus infections could be dramatically lowered in Western cultures if children were not routinely fed cows' milk.

Most cultures in the world are highly allergic to cows' milk, and people in those cultures do not have the enzymes to digest its lactose. Some northern European cultures can tolerate milk to some degree, but for the most part, there is no good reason for milk to be a staple of anybody's diet. It has a poor calcium-to-magnesium ratio, is loaded with fat, and most of our bodies are intolerant of it. Furthermore, dairy cows are forced to exist in intolerably unhealthy conditions and are loaded up with antibiotics and other drugs to compensate. When you drink milk, you are getting dosed with these drugs. The scientist who invented BHT, the controversial hormone that increases milk production in dairy cows, quit his job at Monsanto and is actively campaigning against its use because he believes it is dangerous. The fact that the dairy industry and the FDA have chosen to ignore his warnings and use BHT is evidence enough that profits are more important to them than your health. To add insult to injury, it is illegal for a dairy company *not* using BHT to inform you of that on the label. If you are sure you and your family can tolerate milk, please look for an organic brand.

If you have an infant and can't breast-feed for some reason, look into infant formulas that are not based on cows' milk. Some infants do well on goats' milk. When your infant gets a little older, you can try soy milk and rice milk as alternatives, as long as his or her diet as a whole is well rounded.

Yogurt is another alternative to milk. While it is usually made from cows' milk, the fermenting or culturing process used to make yogurt renders the offending lactose and proteins harmless. Most children will happily eat yogurt. However, I still recommend you not make it an everyday staple of a child's diet—and avoid the flavored yogurts, which are mainly "flavored" with large amounts of sugar. Add your own fruit for variety instead.

Having said all this, what do allergies to cows' milk have to do with hormone balance? When your body is in a chronic, unremitting state of mild inflammation or irritation, as with an allergy, it puts an extra strain on your adrenal glands to provide the anti-inflammatory steroids to combat the allergic reaction. The precursor to these steroids is—you guessed it—progesterone. Just as a deficiency can cause a hormone imbalance, an excessive need for any one hormone throws the others out of balance.

EAT MEAT SPARINGLY

In most of the world, meat is a rare treat. If we in Western, industrialized cultures would think of it more as an occasional food than a main course, we would be much healthier. There is nothing wrong with meat per se, but it's a high-energy, high-fat, concentrated food that most of us, with our sedentary lives, do not need in any large quantity to be healthy and well nourished. Too much protein can cause calcium to be leached from the bones, which contributes greatly to osteoporosis. I suggest you begin to think of meat as a condiment instead of a main dish. Eat smaller portions and start replacing meat dishes with soy and other legumes, fish, and small amounts of fermented dairy products such as yogurt and cheese. Even most vegetables and grains contain small amounts of protein, so getting enough is rarely an issue for most of us. Some grains, such as quinoa and amaranth, are excellent sources of protein.

There is a myth that you need to eat a complete protein, meaning all the essential amino acids, in one meal in order for it to be effective. Believe me, your body is smarter than that. You can eat a grain in the morning and a legume at lunch, and your body will figure out how to put them together to make complete proteins. Again, the key to good nourishment is to eat whole, unrefined, unprocessed foods.

Beef cattle are routinely injected with estrogen pellets to fatten them up for market. This estrogen is still in the meat when it gets to your table. It may be present in very small amounts, but as you have learned from this book, it only takes very small amounts of estrogen to throw your hormones out of balance. When beef cattle were raised on the range and ate grass, their meat was lean and mostly saturated fats. Now they spend the better part of their lives in crowded feedlots being stuffed with corn and soy to increase their weight, and their meat contains odd amalgams of unsaturated and saturated fats. Because the crowded conditions of the feedlots are so unhealthy, they are routinely fed antibiotics, which show up in the meat. Because of this pervasive exposure to antibiotics, more and more bacteria are becoming resistant to them, putting us in the dangerous position of getting an infection and having nothing to fight it with. If you love beef, have it once every week or two as a treat, and try to find a source of range-fed, hormone-free beef. Ask at your supermarket—many are offering "healthy" beef these days, and the manager of the meat department may be willing to order it for you. If you're neutral about beef, I recommend you phase it out of your diet altogether.

Chickens are also raised in extremely crowded, unhealthy, unsanitary conditions and fed all kinds of drugs, including antibiotics, to keep them from getting diseased. Chicken has been touted as a healthy meat, but in truth it contains as much fat as lean beef, and may be even more tainted with drugs and chemicals than beef. Eat chicken sparingly, too, and again, look for free-range, hormone-free chicken.

EAT MORE FISH

Fish are an excellent source of protein, and also contain the omega-3 fatty acids EPA (eicosapentaenoic acid) and DHA (docosahexaenoic acid). These oils have been shown in a number of studies to reduce inflammation, and often also arthritis symptoms. They also help lower cholesterol and thin the blood, reducing your risk of heart attacks and strokes. There is a problem with industrial and pesticide pollution in freshwater fish and fish caught near the coastline in shallow water. The best types to eat are the cold-water, deep-sea fish: salmon, mackerel, herring, sardines, and cod, for example. Albacore tuna is also good, although its flesh tends to accumulate mercury, so it's best not to eat it more than once a week.

EAT MORE FIBER

I've already mentioned the importance of eating plenty of fiber, but it's worth covering in more detail. Lack of fiber causes constipation, which causes all kinds of problems, from gas and indigestion to varicose veins in the legs caused by straining during a bowel movement. Fiber is indigestible plant matter that passes all the way through the digestive tract. On its way through, it has an important cleansing effect, absorbing waste products, including fats, in the large intestine. One of the waste products absorbed by fiber is estrogen. If you don't have enough fiber in your diet, the estrogen may be recycled back into the body. Fiber will also lower cholesterol. People who eat plenty of fiber have lower rates of all types of cancer, especially colon cancer.

The best possible way to get fiber into your diet is to eat whole, unprocessed foods. Whole grains, fresh fruits, vegetables, legumes, and nuts have plenty of fiber. As I said, if your diet is primarily processed foods, please introduce the fiber gradually, so you and your digestive system have time to adjust. You may go through an uncomfortable period of weeks where you are clearing out waste materials that have accumulated in your bowels, but this will pass, and you should be glad to be rid of this waste.

If you want to add even more fiber to your diet, you can take one teaspoon of psyllium seed husk in eight ounces of water or juice every morning. (You need to stir it vigorously and drink it right away.) The pure psyllium you find at your health food store is the same ingredient found in Metamucil and other similar products, without the sweeteners, preservatives, and food colorings.

TAKE SOME VITAMINS

So, do you still need to take vitamins? I recommend it. The reason is that every day we are subjected to environmental pollutants that take a toll on our health, not necessarily in a noticeable way, but over time. Exposure to pesticides and industrial pollutants, car exhaust, various plastics, and additives and preservatives in our foods makes it that much harder for your body to keep up with the job of staying healthy. Taking a few key vitamins can give you the extra health insurance to stay one step ahead. Most vitamins are best taken with meals.

In industrialized cultures where pollution is inescapable, I think everyone should be taking antioxidants daily. Antioxidants will work directly to counteract substances that cause oxidation in the body. Take:

Vitamin C, from 1000 to 2000 milligrams per day in a buffered form. If you have a cold, flu, allergies, arthritis, or virtually any other physical stress on the body, you can take 5000 to 10,000 milligrams per day.

Vitamin E, 400 IU daily. If you know you have been exposed to oxidative stress such as air pollution, take an extra 400 IU.

Quercetin, a powerful antioxidant, is a supplement you can take if you have allergies. It is a yellow bioflavonoid found in many plants and in many of the sulfur-containing foods, such as onions and garlic. There are many bioflavonoids to choose from, but quercetin seems to work the best for allergies. Take 500 milligrams twice daily. You can find it at your local health food store.

If you need some extra support during an illness or an allergy season, add other **bioflavonoid** supplements, such as grapeseed extract and green tea extract. They work with vitamin C to reduce histamines and inflammation. You can also find these bioflavonoids at your local health food store.

The **B vitamins** are important to hormone balance, particularly the adrenal hormones. If you are working to bring your hormones back into balance, I suggest you take a B complex vitamin every day. Be sure it has at least 50 milligrams of vitamin B6. Once you're back in balance, as long as your diet is good, you can stop taking them.

Minerals are very important to hormone balance, especially magnesium. Be sure you're getting a mineral mix in a multivitamin or in a separate multimineral supplement. If you're trying to get your hormones back into balance, take 500 to 1000 milligrams of magnesium in the gluconate or citrate form twice daily. Once your hormones are back to normal, you can reduce the magnesium to once a day and then go off it.

DRINK PLENTY OF CLEAN WATER

Water is an important key to health. Most people in industrialized countries don't drink enough water and are chronically dehydrated. They drink coffee, tea, and soda, but rarely water. Water is nature's inner cleanser. Most of us take a shower daily. Drinking plenty of water is like taking an inner shower. Drinking clean water will help your body clear waste and toxins, it will lower your levels of histamines, which promote allergic reactions and inflammation, and will keep your digestive system functioning smoothly. It will also promote clear, soft skin. Dehydration can create an imbalance of minerals, which will disrupt hormone balance.

Sadly, most water that comes out of your tap is now polluted beyond the point where it is truly safe to drink, and with the addition of chlorine, it generally tastes terrible. Since you can't always trust commercial bottled water to be clean, the best way to get clean water is to put a filter on your kitchen tap. A simple charcoal filter will *not* do the job. Be sure to get a type that filters out chlorine, heavy metals, benzene, and bacteria. You do not have to go to the expense of getting a reverse osmosis system—a ceramic or copper/zinc filter will do the job and takes just a few minutes to install. Check your yellow pages under "water."

GET SOME EXERCISE

Most of our chronic illnesses, such as heart disease, arthritis, and cancer, can be traced to poor diet, lack of exercise, and the obesity caused by lack of exercise. The human body is built for movement. Every system in your body, from your organs, circulatory and lymph systems, to your muscles and bones, performs best for you when it is moved and stretched regularly. This is especially true of hormone balance. Estrogen is made and stored in fatty tissues, so obesity is a major cause of estrogen dominance. Women who are obese also tend to become insulin resistant, which means sugar isn't being removed from the blood and utilized properly. This sets up imbalances in the adrenal glands, which affect the reproductive organs. Your body works as a unit— when one part of it is out of balance, the rest tends to follow.

You don't need to take up jogging or go to the gym to get adequate exercise. For most people, a brisk twenty- to thirty-minute walk every day or so will do the job. I have horses, cows, chickens, geese, cats, and dogs, so I get my exercise doing the chores twice a day. Gardening, raking leaves, mowing the lawn, and shoveling snow are all good exercise. Swimming, bike riding, tennis, and golf also work well. Yoga and the Chinese movement exercises such as tai chi and qi gong are excellent for keeping the body toned and supple. Some people dance, some take aerobics classes, some use exercise videos, others have exercise machines. What's important is to find a form (or forms) of exercise that you enjoy, and then make it a near daily habit. (For most people, planning daily exercise results in actually getting it three to four days a week!)

HOW ARE YOUR ADRENAL GLANDS WORKING?

As you discovered earlier in the book, having healthy adrenal glands is crucial to proper hormone balance.

Lack of adrenal reserve or adrenal exhaustion is caused by chronic, unremitting stress, a common scenario in Western cultures. It can be the cause of debilitating fatigue. The key to healthy adrenal glands is de-stressing your life, getting plenty of sleep, and eating a balanced diet of healthy, whole foods. If your stress is largely mental, I recommend you take up some form of meditation that induces a relaxation response. Exercise can also be relaxing, but if you have adrenal insufficiency, exercise probably makes you even more tired. Since sugar stimulates the adrenals, one of the first steps you can take to support yourself is to eliminate sugar and alcohol from your diet. Progesterone is a precursor to the cortical hormones, so using it may also help significantly. (If you're wondering whether your adrenal glands need some help, please reread Chapter 11, "Hormone Balance, Premenopause Syndrome, and the Adrenal and Thyroid Glands.")

If you have followed the above guidelines for six months and still feel tired most of the time, ask your doctor about using some hydrocortisone for a few months to support your adrenal function. This is a natural form of cortisone (the same molecule as is found in the body), and in small, physiologic doses does not have the side effects of large doses of the synthetic cortisones. In fact, the history of the use of cortisone in the United States is very similar to progesterone: It's a very effective medicine in small doses in its natural form, but since there were no profits to be made from the natural cortisones, the drug companies turned to synthetic versions with all their awful side effects. Research on hydrocortisone was halted and it faded into oblivion as a medicine for the most part. It boggles my mind that millions of people taking large doses of synthetic cortisone may be suffering needlessly because mainstream medicine has forgotten how well the real thing works. If you or your doctor would like to know more about this subject, I highly recommend the book, *The Safe Uses of Cortisone*, by William McK. Jefferies, M.D., F.A.C.P.

DIGESTION

Digestion is an important key to good health and hormone balance. Indigestion interferes with the absorption of nutrients, makes you more susceptible to disease, and can cause food allergies or intolerances. It's nearly impossible to have good overall health without having good digestion as a foundation. If you aren't absorbing your nutrients properly, you won't have the vitamins and minerals necessary to convert one hormone into another.

The most common triggers for indigestion and heartburn are too much fat or fried food, processed meats with nitrates or nitrites in them, too much sugar, alcohol, chocolate, and drugs (especially antibiotics), and stress. If your digestive tract is already irritated, substances such as coffee, citrus fruits, tomato-based foods, and spicy foods will only irritate it more. If you have heartburn, you may be able to cure it simply by eliminating coffee.

If you have heartburn, please do not reach for antacids; they will temporarily suppress the symptoms for an hour or so, but in the long run they will make matters worse. You may even become dependent on them. Antacids also contain aluminum, silicone, sugar, and a long list of dyes and preservatives, none of which will help you and may even harm you. And no matter what the new advertising strategies are, I definitely do not recommend you get extra calcium by chewing on antacid tablets! The side effects of the antacids far outweigh any advantage you might get from the calcium, which is in a poorly absorbed form.

H2 blockers such as Pepcid, Zantac, and Tagamet, which the FDA has allowed to be sold over the counter, are even worse: They suppress the secretion of stomach acid and in many people create a distressingly long list of side effects. They interfere with the absorption of nutrients, especially calcium. Tagamet, one of the best-selling drugs in the United States, has the worst side effects: It can cause breast enlargement in men because it interferes with estrogen metabolism and excretion in the liver. Tagamet enhances the effects of many drugs, which can have deadly side effects. There is absolutely no reason I know of for anyone to take these drugs. They are largely irrevelant in the treatment of ulcers and have way too many side effects to justify their use in something as easily preventable as heartburn. Your stomach acid is also one of your frontline defenses against harmful bacteria. Suppress it, and the rest of your systems have to work overtime to protect you.

In spite of what the makers of Tums, Rolaids, Mylanta, Pepcid, Zantac, and Tagamet would have you believe, heartburn is rarely caused by too much stomach acid. In fact, it's most often caused by *too little* stomach acid. As we age, we tend to produce less stomach acid. Without enough stomach acid, our food isn't properly digested in the stomach and tends to sits there. This is especially true of fatty foods. The longer food sits undigested in the stomach, the better the chance it will be burped back up to irritate the esophagus—the real source of heartburn pain. That feeling of having something stuck in your throat is an almost sure sign of too little stomach acid. Chronic heartburn is usually caused by an esophagus that's irritated by constant exposure to stomach acid.

And by the way, the fancy new term being used in advertisements for heartburn medications, "gastroesophageal reflux," means nothing more than heartburn.

PREVENTING HEARTBURN

- Don't lie down right after you eat. If your esophageal muscle is already too relaxed or weak, your semidigested meal will escape back up your throat.
- Eat small meals and chew your food thoroughly. Overeating and eating on the run are two of the most common causes of heartburn.
- Obesity can cause heartburn.
- If you drink a lot of alcohol, cutting down (no more than two drinks daily) will almost certainly help long-term,

and abstaining while you have symptoms will make healing much faster.

- If you have a sweet tooth, that could be the culprit. For
  some reason, chocolate is particularly aggravating to
  many people.
- Many prescription medications cause heartburn. Ask your
  doctor or pharmacist if you're taking a drug that causes
  heartburn.
- In case you need another reason to give up cigarettes, stop
  smoking and your heartburn may disappear. Nicotine
  relaxes the sphincter muscle that separates the esophagus
  from the stomach, allowing stomach acid to reflux
  (burp) up.
- Stress greatly aggravates heartburn by suppressing stomach acid.

Most people with chronic heartburn, especially those over the
age of 50, have low levels of hydrochloric acid (HCl), the main
digestive acid in the stomach. The most common symptoms of a
stomach acid deficiency show up after eating, in the form of
heartburn, belching, bloating, or a heavy feeling. If you feel that
most of your meal is still in your stomach more than 45 minutes
after eating a normal meal, your stomach is working inefficiently.
One way to stimulate your digestive juices is to drink a glass of
water half an hour before eating. Other people swear by a table-
spoon of apple cider vinegar in one-third of a cup of water before
a meal. Vinegar is highly acidic and may provide your stomach
with enough acidity for quick, easy digestion.

If none of the other heartburn prevention and treatment sug-
gestions work, you can try taking betaine hydrochloride (HCl)
supplements. But please don't take vinegar or start HCl supplements while you have an active case of heartburn. This will only
irritate your esophagus even more. Wait until you feel better, then
try taking one tablet with food. You can increase your dose up to

two to three tablets per meal, but if you get a burning feeling in your stomach, you're taking too much. You can buy HCl supplements at health food stores and at some pharmacies.

TAKING CARE OF THE LARGE INTESTINE: PROBIOTICS

During the last stages of digestion in the large intestine and colon, what was once food is now mostly waste products, fiber, and water. The colon, in contrast to the germ-free stomach, is heavily populated with both "good" and "bad" bacteria. In a healthy system, the "good" bacteria run the show in the colon, keeping the "bad" bacteria under control. Probiotics are the "good" bacteria found in your intestines as well as other parts of the body, such as the mouth, the urinary tract, and the vagina. Your overall health is closely tied to the health of these bacteria. If they are sick, often so are you. Along with our digestive enzymes, they play a major role in digesting food and moving it out of the body.

The three most common families of friendly bacteria are called *lactobacillus acidophilus, lactobacillus bulgaricus,* and *bifidobacterium bifidum.* These versatile bugs change and adapt rapidly, depending upon geographic location, individual biochemistry, and what types of unfriendly bacteria are invading the body at the moment. Probiotics are the ultimate antibiotics, elegantly crafted by nature to fight off unfriendly bacteria without killing the friendly ones. It's simple—take care of your friendly bacteria and they will take care of you.

Probiotics play other roles as well: Your immune system depends on them; they manufacture the B vitamins, which play a major role in adrenal hormone production; they reduce cholesterol and help keep all your hormones in balance.

The surest way to get in trouble with your friendly bacteria is to take antibiotics, which kill the friendly bacteria along with the unfriendly ones. Always follow antibiotic treatment with at least two weeks of probiotics. Other factors are a poor diet, stress, and poor digestion in the stomach and small intestine. Probiotics also decline as we age, so if you're having digestive problems or working to bring your hormones back into balance, it's important to add probiotic supplements to your diet or eat yogurt with *live cultures* (check the label) daily. Many supermarkets and health food stores also sell acidophilus, a milk product containing live cultures. Probiotics are "alive" and have a relatively short shelf life of a few months. If you want to try probiotic supplements, buy the refrigerated capsules. You can find them at your health food store.

SPECIAL FOODS FOR HORMONE BALANCE

There are literally thousands of plants that contain sterols, and many vegetables are included in that category. Plant sterols are close relatives of human steroid hormones. In some cases your body will use the sterols to balance your hormones by filling hormone receptors. For example, the phytoestrogens found in soybeans can take up estrogen receptors, but have only very weak, if any, actual estrogenic activity in your body. Thus eating soy can be an indirect way of reducing estrogen effects by occupying your estrogen receptors with something besides estrogen itself.

The sterol in soy called diosgenin is actually used commercially to manufacture many types of pharmaceutical hormone products, including progesterone, DHEA, estrogen, testosterone, and the cortisones. Diosgenin's molecular configuration makes it a convenient laboratory precursor to human steroid hormones. The final product of this laboratory processing produces molecules identical to the ones found in the human body and thus, even though they are manufactured in the laboratory, we can call them natural hormones. It is unfortunate that the pharmaceutical companies then change the natural molecules to create synthetic drugs not found in nature to increase their profits at the expense of your health.

Although we can create natural human steroid hormones from diosgenin in the laboratory, technically speaking there are no biochemical pathways in the body for breaking down diosgenin into progesterone, DHEA, estrogen, testosterone, and the cortisones.

Studies on diosgenin's activity in the human body have failed to show any effect of raising hormone levels, but it is intriguing that the one action diosgenin does sometimes have is to lower total cholesterol levels. We also know that the Japanese, whose diet is high in soy, have a far lower rate of breast and prostate cancer than we do in Western industrialized cultures, and when they move to America and change their diet, their rate of breast and prostate cancer matches ours. I wouldn't, however, use this as a reason to run out and eat soy three times a day. The Japanese have one of the highest rates of stomach cancer in the world, and this may have something to do with the fact that soy is a protease inhibitor—that is, it inhibits the enzyme protease, which is responsible for breaking down protein in the digestive tract. Their high stomach cancer rate may also have to do with the fact that they eat a lot of salted and pickled foods, or that they live in very densely populated cities. We don't know.

I do recommend that you eat plenty of fresh vegetables to take advantage of the presence of plant sterols, and certainly do begin to incorporate soy into your diet a few times a week. You can use soy milk in place of cows' milk, you can use tofu and tempeh in place of meat, and you can make a simple, quick, nutritious soup from miso, which is fermented soybean paste. If you're not familiar with these foods, you can introduce yourself to them through one of the excellent natural foods cookbooks listed in the Recommended Reading section at the back of the book. As with all new foods, introduce them slowly, in small portions, to give your body time to adapt.

HERBS FOR HORMONE BALANCE

Although I did not use herbs in my medical practice because I wasn't trained in their proper use, I'm sure they have a place in treating hormone imbalances. I have spoken to a number of physicians and other health care practitioners who have successfully used herbs to help their patients balance their hormones, in conjunction with a balanced diet, some vitamin and mineral supplements, and exercise. Some herbs contain relatively high levels of plant sterols, and others contain a combination of substances that seem to help balance hormones by bringing the whole body into better balance.

Overall, herbal tinctures (the herb extracted and preserved in a liquid form with alcohol) seem to work better than capsules or tablets, and tinctures made from the fresh plant seem to be preferable to the dried plant.

Although herbs are generally safer and gentler than pharmaceutical drugs in their actions, they should be used only as prescribed. Taking high doses of any medicine can be harmful. Please be sensible and moderate in your use of herbs. None of these herbs should be used by pregnant women, except under the supervision of a health care practitioner experienced in their use. As you will discover as you read about these herbs, the fact that they contain plant sterols doesn't necessarily mean they all have the same effect. For example, fenugreek can stimulate a miscarriage, while unicorn root can prevent one. They can also have very different effects on different people. If you want to use herbs to help balance your hormones, I recommend you work with an experienced herbalist, such as a Chinese medicine doctor or a naturopathic doctor. I am including the following list of herbs more to clear up some of the misconceptions about them than to provide a guide for using them.

Dong quai or angelica (*Angelica sinensis, Angelical polymorpha*) might best be called a woman's tonic. We have recently rediscovered it in the West thanks to the Chinese, who use it extensively in their medicine. Contrary to popular opinion, Dong quai does not contain any estrogen or phytoestrogens, or have any type of estrogenic activity. What it does do is affect the uterine muscles by contracting or relaxing them, enhances metabolism, improves liver function (which improves the excretion of hormones), aids in the utilization of vitamin E, stabilizes heart rhythm, lowers blood pressure by dilating blood vessels, and has a mild sedative activity. Overall, Dong quai might best be labeled an adaptogen, as ginseng is, meaning it tends to bring the entire organism into greater balance. The Chinese use it to bring on menstrual periods, as a tonic for women who have just given birth, as a mild sedative, and for stomachaches.

Angelica archangelica is another type of angelica, in a different plant family (*Apiaceae*) from the Dong quai angelica (*Umbelliferae*), which does appear to have some hormonal activity. It is also known as masterwort. This plant is more a stimulant than a sedative and in folklore is used to bring on menstrual periods.

Fenugreek (*Trigonella foenum-graecum*) is best known as an herbal tea with a maple syrup–like flavor. Fenugreek seeds contain plant sterols, including diosgenin, in relatively large amounts. Fenugreek has oxytocin-like properties, which means it can induce uterine contractions. This can be helpful when a menstrual period is late, but it could theoretically end a pregnancy. Fenugreek also lowers blood sugar and cholesterol, and the seeds, when eaten, can act as a laxative.

Unicorn root (*Aletris farinosa*) is not well researched, but we do know it contains a form of diosgenin and has some type of hormonal activity. Herbalists use it to alleviate menopausal symptoms, to prevent miscarriage, and to stimulate menstrual flow, which seems contradictory, but the adaptogenic herbs seem to work by bringing what is out of balance into balance. Since unicorn root is one of the most popular menopausal herbs, it may be worth trying, especially in combination with other herbs.

Sarsaparilla (*Smilax spp.*) used to be sold as a soda or tonic that was supposed to "cleanse the blood" and cure whatever ailed you. It does contain plant sterols called "saponins," and in fact a component of it, called "sarsasapogenin," has a structural similarity to some of the human steroid hormones. Male athletes have tried using it as a steroid replacement, but I don't know of any studies showing it actually worked. According to herbalist Michael Moore, it is a gentle adrenocortical stimulant, which could make it useful for balancing hormones, particularly if there is adrenal insufficiency.

Licorice (*Glycyrrhiza glabra and uralensis*) is said to be the most common ingredient in Chinese herbal formulas. We know it works well in the treatment of ulcers, probably by encouraging the production of the protective mucosa that lines the stomach. It also has hormonal effects that seem to vary from person to person. The Chinese use licorice extensively to treat any type of adrenal insufficiency. A component of licorice called "glycyrrhizin," if taken in large doses over a long period of time, can raise blood pressure by causing sodium retention and potassium loss. Many licorice tinctures come degly-cyrrhizinized, thus eliminating that concern, but also possibly eliminating many of the therapeutic effects they might have in balancing hormones.

Wild yam (*Dioscorea villosa*) was and still is used extensively by pharmaceutical companies to manufacture steroid hormones from its diosgenin, including pregnenolone, progesterone, DHEA, estrogen, testosterone, and the cortisones. It is this use that has caused the progesterone in many progesterone creams to be labeled "wild yam extract." This, unfortunately, has become misleading, as companies seeking to jump onto the progesterone bandwagon have (out of ignorance or the desire for profit) added diosgenin to a cream, and claim it does the same thing as progesterone. Diosgenin does *not* equal progesterone.

Do not use creams that say "wild yam extract" for progesterone unless you know for sure they contain progesterone. If you call the company that makes the cream, they should be able to tell you exactly how much progesterone is in the cream. If they can't or they hem and haw about whether there is progesterone in the cream, don't buy the product. There are plenty of reputable progesterone products on the market, which are listed on page 334.

HORMONE BALANCE FOR CHILDREN AND TEENS

The secret to hormone balance and later arrival of puberty in teenagers is pretty much the same as the secret to hormone balance throughout life: good nutrition and exercise. The ups and downs of adolescent hormones can often be minimized with a healthy lifestyle. But perhaps the biggest threat to the hormone balance of our children is the contamination of meat with estrogen.

Estrogen is the hormone that stimulates the growth of female characteristics at puberty. Early puberty results in a longer lifetime exposure to estrogen produced by the ovaries, thus increasing cancer risk. It also appears to lead to earlier follicle burnout and anovulatory cycles, starting as early as the midthirties for many women. Just a generation or two ago, teenage girls didn't reach puberty until their late teens. Now they may start menstruating as early as 11 or 12 years old. We have come to think of this as normal. It's not. My suspicion is that this early onset of puberty is caused by exposure to the estrogens and xenoestrogens so prevalent in every part of our environment, from our meat supply to the air we breathe.

Meat is sold by the pound, so meat farmers do everything possible to fatten up their livestock before they're sent to market. Feeding estrogen-like hormones to livestock is by far the most effective, quickest, and cheapest way to fatten them up. In the 1970s and 1980s in Puerto Rico, there was an epidemic of early puberty in girls as young as a year old and even in young boys who developed breasts, caused by meat and dairy products containing high levels of estrogen. The use of estrogen-like hormones in livestock is slightly better regulated in the United States, but it is still very much in use and frequently abused.

DES (diethylstilbestrol), a type of synthetic estrogen, was the first hormone used by the meat industry to fatten up livestock until it was discovered that it causes cancer even in extremely minute amounts.

Hormones are used throughout the meat industry in nearly all Western industrialized countries. Until we wake up to the dramatic effect this practice is having on our hormones, the safest approach to hormone balance is to minimize your children's meat consumption or spend a little extra money on hormone-free meat. (Even with hormone-free meat, I recommend you learn to use it as a condiment instead of a main dish because of its high fat content.)

Another reason to keep meat consumption low is that too much protein contributes to osteoporosis. Too much protein creates an acidic condition in the body that has to be buffered with calcium before it can be excreted in the urine. If not enough calcium is available for this buffering process, it will be pulled from the bones. Childhood and adolescence are times to be building bone, not losing it!

Soda pop is one of the biggest threats to the long-term health and well-being of your children. It contains phosphorous, an acidic substance that also leaches calcium from the bones. Even a reasonably good diet won't be able to keep up with the loss of bone caused by heavy soda consumption. Young girls who drink a lot of soda are setting themselves up for osteoporosis later in life. Soda also contains an enormous amount of sugar. For example, one can of Coke contains nine teaspoons of sugar. Dumping nine teaspoons of sugar into your body is a setup for wildly fluctuating blood sugar, weight gain, insulin resistance, and adrenal fatigue—a perfect setup for hormone imbalances! Just as bad are the diet sodas with aspartame, a synthetic chemical containing substances called excitotoxins, which are known to cause brain damage and may contribute to hyperactivity, learning disabilities, and Alzheimer's.

As with adults, good nutrition for children and adolescents means eating a plant-based diet with meat used sparingly. Children and teens can afford to eat more fat in their diet than adults, say up to 30 percent, but certainly not the 40 to 50 percent so common among that age group. Encourage your kids to resist the temptation to eat junk foods. When they crave fat, give them hormone-free beef or chicken, or vegetables stir-fried in a small amount of unrefined coconut oil. When they crave salty foods, give them pop-corn, corn chips (without added oil), or rice cakes. When they crave sweets, give them fruit, so they'll get some fiber with their sugar. If you do this at home and let them know why in a friendly way, they will be more inclined to make healthy eating decisions when they're out with friends.

After 30 years in family practice, I would say exercise is one of the most important factors in navigating successfully through the teen years. I would encourage parents of teenagers to make some sort of after-school exercise mandatory to the extent that is possible. It doesn't matter whether it's a team sport, horseback riding, ice skating, gymnastics, or aikido, just so they're active, involved, and moving. This is the best way I know to channel adolescent energy in a positive way and maintain health and hormone balance. Naturally, if you allow them to choose their own sport, they're much more likely to attend without pressure.

In my own experience, I encouraged children, including my own, to take up noncontact sports. I have seen too many injuries from football, for instance. Sport exercise should be fun, and not a painful experience that risks parental criticism or even rejection.

Supplements for Children and Teens

If you have teens with acne, depression, and other signs of extreme hormone swings, the first step is correcting their diet to avoid milk, meat, and refined foods in favor of fresh, relatively unprocessed plant-based foods, such as whole grains, more vegetables, legumes, and fresh fruit. In this manner they will be avoiding xenoestrogens and other foreign chemicals added to processed foods, and they will be receiving a full complement of important nutrients that are missing in animal products and refined or processed foods. Supplementation with antioxidants such as vitamin C (500 milligrams) and vitamin E (100 milligrams) will help buffer against environmental pollutants. Carrots are always in season and provide good levels of beta-carotene, as are sweet potatoes, butternut squash, and deep green leafy vegetables such as kale, spinach, and chard.

HORMONE BALANCE FOR YOUNG WOMEN

The biggest threat to hormone balance in young women is doctors who insist on giving them birth control pills. There is a mountain of evidence showing that birth control pills cause numerous and serious health problems, including depression, headaches, nausea, fluid retention, high cholesterol, high triglyceride levels, liver disease, urinary tract infections, all of the estrogen dominance symptoms, all of the side effects caused by the progestins, and most dangerous of all, blood clots leading to pulmonary embolisms (blood clots in the lungs) and strokes. These dangers to individual women are swept under the carpet for the "higher good" of reducing the population, but you can bet that a drug that dangerous would never be given to men on such a wide scale.

I strongly urge parents to educate their daughters about the delicacy of hormonal balance, and discourage the use of hormonal contraceptives of *any* kind. A good "rite of passage" book for teenage girls who have begun to menstruate is the book, *The New Our Bodies, Ourselves,* by the Boston Women's Health Collective. This book gives accurate, detailed information about the pros and cons of various methods of birth control, as well as about relationships, sexuality, sexually transmitted diseases, pregnancy, and so forth. It's a straightforward, no-nonsense sourcebook for women, especially young women with questions about their newly developing bodies.

Unfortunately, intellectual knowledge of hormones is of little import when compared to the primary drives activated by pubertal hormones. Most often the young learn from each other rather than from parental figures, who are regarded by the young as basically sexless and unable to understand what they are going through. I recall a woman and her teenage daughter arriving at my office, the mother angry at the school for showing an educational movie about sex and pregnancy. As it happened, the daughter had fainted during the showing of the movie, and the mother had been called to take the daughter to be medically examined. The mother was upset that the daughter had been exposed to such explicit sexual knowledge at such a tender age. I turned to the daughter and asked her what it was about the movie that had upset her so. After a bit of hemming and hawing, she admitted that, in watching the movie, she realized that her activities with her boyfriend might have made her pregnant. At that, the mother almost fainted herself! She had no idea her daughter was no longer a child but a young woman and, as such, needed all the education she could get about sexual matters. The mother later became an ardent advocate of even earlier school sex education.

Supplements for Young Women

Vitamin needs for young women are about the same as for teens. A basic multivitamin with plenty of antioxidants (500 milligrams of vitamin C, 200 IU of vitamin E) should be enough to provide some buffer against environmental pollutants, providing their diet is reasonable and they're getting some exercise.

HORMONE BALANCE FOR PREMENOPAUSAL WOMEN

The biggest threat to the hormone balance of premenopausal women is doctors who want to castrate them, an operation otherwise known as a hysterectomy. I see no reason for any woman to have a hysterectomy unless she has cancer. (See Chapter 16 for details.) The most common reason women are talked into having a hysterectomy is bleeding caused by uterine fibroids. As you'll remember, uterine fibroids can be reduced in size to the point where they are harmless with the use of progesterone. After menopause they usually disappear altogether.

Women may begin to have signs of menopause as early as their midthirties, in the form of anovulatory cycles that begin to create estrogen dominance and all its myriad symptoms, such as weight gain, fatigue, depression, mood swings, fluid retention, unstable blood sugar, low thyroid symptoms, fibrocystic breasts, and uterine fibroids. Although menstrual periods will continue even when there is no ovulation, they may be farther apart, or heavier, or lighter. Adrenal insufficiency caused by a stressful lifestyle may exacerbate symptoms of estrogen dominance. Since a woman must ovulate to become pregnant, infertility can also be a problem for women trying to get pregnant at this age. I suspect a lot of chronic fatigue syndrome is really hormonal mayhem caused by a combination of estrogen dominance and adrenal insufficiency.

If you are experiencing these symptoms in your midthirties, you have a number of options. Your first course of action should be to examine your lifestyle, and then review the hormone balance program above. If you are eating poorly, not drinking enough water, not exercising, and stressed out, there isn't a magic pill or cream to heal that! Only you can heal that. Taking care of your own health should be your top priority. When you do, you will be amazed at how many other parts of your life begin to come into balance.

If you are scientifically minded, you can pay a visit to your doctor and ask to have your hormone levels tested. The emerging technique of testing saliva hormone levels will probably be of great usefulness here.

Another option is simply to try using some progesterone cream from day 12 to 26 of your cycle to find out if that helps or relieves your symptoms. Many women have told me that their body seems to breathe a sigh of relief after only one or two days using the cream, and their symptoms start to disappear. Some women lose five pounds of water weight after only a week or two of using progesterone. For others, it takes weeks or even up to two months to start noticing positive changes. Some women initially have unpleasant symptoms of estrogen dominance, such as breast tenderness, exaggerated because the progesterone temporarily sensitizes their estrogen receptors. This usually disappears after a week or two. When you begin using progesterone, I suggest you keep a brief daily journal for at least three months to track your physical, emotional, and mental health.

As I mentioned, if you are using progesterone and still have signs of adrenal insufficiency (see Chapter 11), consider using some low-dose hydrocortisone for a while. As I've explained, your doctor is likely to panic when you mention cortisone because there is such a strong mindset that it is harmful, which it is when you use the synthetic versions or high doses. If your doctor panics, ask him or her to read this book, or William Jefferies's book, *The Safe Uses of Cortisone.*

Sometimes using thyroid hormone will help bring things back into balance, too, although in the past few years I think thyroid has been used too often, when all that is needed is some basic hormone balance. If your doctor does decide you could use some thyroid hormone, please reread Chapter 11 on hormone balance and the thyroid.

If you have a petite build, small bones, and a history of osteoporosis in your family, I recommend you get a bone density test in your late thirties. If you have already begun losing bone density, start using progesterone cream immediately. (See page 315 for Dr. Lee's Osteoporosis Treatment Program.)

Supplements for Premenopausal Women

If you are eating good, nourishing, whole foods, drinking plenty of clean water, getting some exercise, and have good digestion, your need for vitamins should be minimal.

If your hormones are out of balance, take:

- A vitamin B complex that includes 50 milligrams of vitamin B6
- Vitamin C, 1000 milligrams twice daily, up to 5000 to 10,000 milligrams daily, in a buffered form
- Vitamin E, 400 IU daily, up to 800 IU daily
- Magnesium, 500 milligrams at bedtime

When your hormones are back in balance, you can try cutting back to just the antioxidants: Vitamin C, at least 1000 milligrams daily, and vitamin E, 400 IU daily.

HORMONE BALANCE FOR MENOPAUSAL WOMEN

The biggest threat to the hormone balance of menopausal women is doctors who want to put them on HRT (hormone replacement therapy). Be wary of another pattern I've been hearing about from women and their doctors: Women in their late forties or early fifties pay a visit to their doctor, who insists they begin taking HRT. The woman complies and returns a year later for a Pap test, which shows abnormal tissue growth. The doctor does not tell the woman that this tissue growth may well be caused by the HRT, but does tell her she has a "precancerous" condition and must have a hysterectomy right away. After the hysterectomy, she is once again put on HRT. What's wrong with this picture?

First of all, I don't know of any reason why any woman should be subjected to synthetic hormones. The natural hormones are available and are much safer and freer of side effects. Secondly, there is only a very small percentage of women who ever need estrogen supplementation, and then they may only need some vaginal cream to treat vaginal dryness. Most women go through menopause just fine, thank you, and, at most, need some progesterone. The third thing wrong with this picture is that the "precancerous" changes in tissue that show up on a Pap smear when a woman is on HRT or is estrogen dominant will, in all likelihood, disappear after a few months of taking progesterone. This tissue growth is directly caused by estrogen, is very slow-growing, and poses no short-term threat. There is no reason to panic or rush into surgery.

If you are experiencing hot flashes and vaginal dryness or any of the symptoms of estrogen dominance, try some progesterone cream. If that doesn't help, try a small amount of estrogen (either estrone or estriol vaginal cream) for a few months, and then taper it off very gradually over another two months. Chances are, you'll only need to take the estrogen for a few months to a year before your hormones begin to come into balance. Menopausal symptoms are caused not so much by declining hormone levels as by an *abrupt* drop in hormones. Most severe so-called menopause symptoms are caused by surgically induced menopause in the form of a hysterectomy.

As we age, our digestion is not as efficient, and we don't absorb nutrients as well as we used to. For this reason I emphasize taking good care of your digestion by eating plenty of fiber and either eating yogurt regularly or taking acidophilus supplements to provide "friendly" bacteria to your intestines.

A high percentage of older women are at risk for osteoporosis. After a good diet and exercise, progesterone is by far the best way to prevent or reverse osteoporosis.

Supplements for Menopausal Women

If you are eating good, nourishing, whole foods, drinking plenty of clean water, getting some exercise, and have good digestion, your need for vitamins should be minimal. However, older people have less efficient digestive systems; and in addition, it's helpful to protect against environmental pollutants with antioxidants. If you are at risk for osteoporosis, see Dr. Lee's Osteoporosis Treatment Program below. Otherwise, take:

- A multivitamin; those over the age of 70 might want to consider taking a powdered vitamin that is mixed with juice, such as All-One (made by All One People, Santa Barbara, CA). These are easier to absorb than tablets
- Vitamin C, 1000 milligrams twice daily, up to 5000 to 10,000 milligrams daily, in a buffered form
- Vitamin E, 400 IU, up to 800 IU daily
- Magnesium, 500 milligrams at bedtime; if you have leg cramps at night, try taking a calcium/magnesium supplement before bed with a little yogurt

DR. LEE'S OSTEOPOROSIS TREATMENT PROGRAM

Diet	Low-protein diet with leafy greens, legumes, and whole grains emphasized. Avoid all sodas. Limit alcohol use.
Vitamin D	350 to 400 IU daily

Vitamin C	2000 milligrams a day in divided doses
Beta-carotene	15 milligrams a day
Vitamin B6	50 milligrams a day
Zinc	15 to 30 milligrams a day
Magnesium	300 to 500 milligrams a day
Calcium	800 to 1000 milligrams a day, mostly by diet (may use one 300-milligram supplement per day)
Progesterone	3% cream applied at bedtime daily, 21 days a month if postmenopausal, or the two weeks before menses if not menopausal. Use 1 to 2 ounces a month. Dose may be reduced later depending on serial BMD results.
Estrogen	Indicated for vaginal dryness or hot flashes in post-menopausal women. If not medically contraindicated, may use low-dose (0.3 to 0.625 milligrams a day) of estriol for three weeks a month. Often not needed.
Exercise	Twenty minutes daily or one-half hour three times a week. Exercise that brings out a little sweat builds bones better than lighter exercise. Find exercise that's fun to do.

No cigarette smoking.

Report **any** occurrence of vaginal bleeding to your doctor.

For details of this program, please refer to Chapter 12, "Hormone Balance and Osteoporosis" (page 150).

THE HORMONE BALANCE PROGRAM AT A GLANCE

- If you are smoking, quit—now.
- Keep alcohol consumption to two drinks a day or less.
- Eat whole, fresh, preferably organic foods and avoid refined and processed foods, additives, preservatives, and colorings.
- Drink plenty of clean water and avoid soda pop.
- Keep fat consumption to 20 to 25 percent of your calorie intake.
- Emphasize olive oil and avoid hydrogenated oils and most vegetable oils.
- Eat a plant-based diet, emphasizing plenty of fresh, preferably organic vegetables, whole grains, legumes, nuts, and fruit.
- Eat small portions of meat (including beef, pork, and chicken) no more than two to three times a week.
- Eat modest servings of eggs, yogurt, and deep-sea, cold-water ocean fish four to five times a week.
- Take some antioxidant vitamins and if you're over 50, take a multivitamin as well.
- Get some moderate exercise, preferably every day, but at least three times a week.
- Keep your digestion working well by eating plenty of fiber, and use probiotics (acidophilus) if necessary.
- Use some progesterone cream if necessary.
- Avoid doctors who want to put you on synthetic HRT or take out your uterus if they won't try natural, noninvasive options with no side effects first.

Chapter 20

COMMONLY ASKED QUESTIONS ABOUT USING NATURAL PROGESTERONE

After giving hundreds of talks around the world about progesterone, I've found that the same questions tend to come up over and over again. While all these questions have been thoroughly answered in the preceding chapters, I hope this list of questions and succinct answers will provide a useful refresher and guide.

Q: How long should I stay on progesterone supplementation?

A: Since progesterone has so many positive benefits and no known side effects, there is no reason to discontinue it. I tell women to continue until age 96 and then we'll reevaluate.

Q: How do I know how much progesterone to use?

A: The goal is to restore normal physiologic progesterone levels for at least two to three weeks a month. An ovulating woman makes about 20 to 24 milligrams a day for about 12 days each month after ovulation, or about 240 milligrams a month. Let's say a progesterone cream supplies 480 milligrams of progesterone per ounce (960 milligrams per two-ounce jar). Even at 50-percent absorption, one ounce of cream used up over two to three weeks will supply 240 milligrams a month, the same amount as an ovulating woman.

If a woman has not been making progesterone for a number of years (often starting five to 10 years before actual menopause), her body-fat progesterone is probably very low. Since progesterone is fat-soluble, it is likely that during the first month or so, much of the progesterone that is absorbed will be taken up by body fat, resulting in lower blood levels initially. For these women, I recommend using two ounces (one jar) of the cream each month for the first two months. After that, one ounce (one-half a jar) should be a sufficient monthly dose. Many postmenopausal women do well on one-third of a jar each month.

Since prevention or reversal of osteoporosis is a goal of progesterone usage, serial lumbar bone mineral density (BMD) tests are helpful. If the BMD rises on one-half a jar per month for 10 to 12 months, then one knows that the progesterone dosage is sufficient. If you are using a full jar per month and observe good BMD results, you can reduce to one-half a jar per month and recheck the BMD in another year. Since individual needs vary, the correct dose is the dose that works.

If BMD is low and does not improve after 10 to 12 months of progesterone usage at the levels described above, the cause of the failure to improve is probably some other factor in bone building, such as diet, lack of exercise, nutritional deficiency, or taking a medication that causes bone loss, such as an antacid. All the various factors described in Chapter 12 on osteoporosis would then need to be reevaluated.

Q: But shouldn't I be taking estrogen for my heart?
A: Despite the advertising, the cardiovascular protection bene-

fit of estrogen supplementation is still questionable. Estrogen does appear to lower total cholesterol and raise HDL cholesterol modestly. But it is not clear that this reduces the risk of heart mortality per se, as shown by the recent report titled "Serum Total Cholesterol and Long-Term Coronary Heart Disease (CHD) Mortality in Different Cultures," by W. M. Monique Vershuren, and published in *JAMA* (*Journal of the American Medical Association*). The authors concluded that other factors, such as diet and antioxidants, are probably more important in heart disease prevention.

In the several studies that claim to show reduction in heart deaths in estrogen-taking women, there are differences in other heart risk factors between the test group and the control group. In other words, the study compared apples with oranges. In addition, in the most prominent study (Nurses' Questionnaire Study), the risk of "ischemic" stroke (i.e., clot-caused) was significantly higher in the estrogen-taking nurses.

Remember, other factors are known to reduce heart disease risks significantly. These factors include a plant-based diet (avoiding red meat and dairy products, especially milk), eating more seafood, taking antioxidant vitamins such as E, beta-carotene, and C, and mineral supplements such as magnesium, potassium, and selenium. Modest amounts of alcohol and eggs do not increase heart risk.

The increased risk of heart disease after menopause may be the result of progesterone deficiency rather than estrogen deficiency. Heart disease risk is highly variable when different cultures are examined, yet all women experience menopause.

Over the past 15 years, I have been struck by the fact that my patients on progesterone supplementation (and without estrogen supplements) have been remarkably free of heart disease. Clearly there are other factors involved. The role of estrogen per se is still questionable.

Q: Who should use estrogen supplements?

A: Estrogen works especially well for hot flashes and vaginal dryness. These symptoms can be taken as a sign of estrogen deficiency. However, because progesterone is a biochemical precursor to estrogen, it alone is often sufficient to restore estrogen levels to normal and eliminate these symptoms. If a three-month trial of progesterone plus proper diet and supplements of magnesium and B6 do not relieve hot flashes or vaginal dryness, then low-dose *natural* estrogen may be helpful. (Estrogen is not recommended in those women with a history of breast or uterine cancer, obesity, diabetes, or a history of clotting or vascular disorders.) If used for hot flashes, find the lowest dose of estrogen that works. If vaginal dryness is the problem, I usually recommend vaginal gels or creams containing estrone or estriol. Often, a small dose applied in the vagina only twice a week, three weeks a month, will do wonders. Otherwise, I'm not sure of any reason to use estrogen.

Q: I'm still having periods, but I have problems with hot flashes, water retention, poor sleep, and mood swings. What is wrong with me?

A: During the years before actual menopause, estrogen may be decreasing slightly and, more often, ovulation has ceased or is rare. Without ovulation, progesterone production is essentially zero, and estrogen receptors become less sensitive to the estrogen still being made. You are actually estrogen dominant. Your doctor, however, will probably prescribe estrogen, but the results are only partially effective and many of the problems, such as fluid retention, become worse. When a synthetic progestin is added, the results are usually not good because progestins are not the same as natural progesterone and also cause undesirable side effects. The best treatment is a plant-based diet, vitamin E, magnesium, and vitamin B6 supplements, plus natural progesterone. In these cases, progesterone can be added during the "luteal" phase, that is, from day 12 (ovulation time) to day 26 (48 hours before the expected period).

Q: My periods are sometimes scant, sometimes heavy, and sometimes come early or late. What should I do?

A: Irregular periods in the years before menopause are another sign that menopause is approaching, and you are most probably deficient in progesterone due to not ovulating every month. Remember, shedding of the bloody endometrial lining is triggered primarily by the fall of progesterone levels 12 days or so after ovulation. If you are not ovulating, you are not making much progesterone, and therefore there will be no fall of progesterone to trigger a proper shedding. Follow the advice of the previous question for at least three cycles and your periods should become more regular again.

Q: I'm 43 years old and still having periods, but I've lost interest in sex. What's wrong?

A: Libido (the desire for sex) is mistakenly thought by most doctors to come from estrogen. The fact that you are still having periods means you are making plenty of estrogen. But you are most probably low in progesterone. Progesterone is an important factor in libido. Testosterone also improves libido. Since most doctors are unaware of this role of progesterone, some are tempted to give women testosterone for their flagging libido. However, this choice is less desirable because of the masculinizing effects of testosterone. The more desirable choice is natural progesterone. Follow the advice of the two previous questions and your libido will most probably return to normal. Don't worry; you will not become a sex maniac—the guy across the room will just become a little better-looking, that's all.

Q: Help! My hair is falling out by the handful.

A: When progesterone levels fall as a result of ovarian follicle failure (lack of ovulation), the body responds by increasing its production of the adrenal cortical steroid, androstenedione, an alternative precursor for the production of other adrenal cortical hormones. Androstenedione conveys some androgenic (male-like) properties, in this case, male pattern hair loss. When progesterone levels are raised by progesterone supplements, the androstenedione level will gradually fall, and your normal hair growth will eventually resume. Since hair growth is a slow process, it may take four to six months for the effects to become apparent.

Q: My sister developed breast cancer when she was 45 and still menstruating. I'm now 43 and my periods are changing. What should I do?

A: The actual causes of breast cancer are still largely unknown, but most authorities agree that estrogen is at least a promoter of breast cancer. In industrialized countries, it has become epidemic that progesterone deficiency and estrogen dominance among women occur during their midthirties. (This is probably due to xenobiotic [petrochemical] toxins affecting ovary development during the embryo stage.) Estrogen dominance increases the risk of breast cancer. To prevent breast cancer, it is wise to follow a plant-based diet to avoid xenoestrogens in red meat and dairy foods, and to supplement with natural progesterone. Avoid synthetic progestins; they may increase breast cancer risk, whereas natural progesterone protects against breast cancer.

Q: My own doctor doesn't seem to know much about natural progesterone. What should I do?

A: Tell your doctor that it's your body and you have the right to choose what to do for it, and point out that natural progesterone is available without prescription. Tell your doctor that whether he or she knows much about it or not, you plan to use natural progesterone. Ask your doctor to follow along with you, that's all. If you like your doctor, it's better to train him/her than to go doctor-shopping. If you're not particularly pleased with your doctor, you always have the option of looking for another one who is more open-minded. You can also give your doctor a copy of this book or my book written for doctors, *Natural Progesterone: the Multiple Roles of a Remarkable Hormone.* (See the Resources section on page 334 for more information.)

Q: What progesterone cream should I use?

A: Use a progesterone cream that contains at least 400 milligrams of progesterone per ounce. (See the report on page 271 on levels of progesterone in commercial creams and oils.) There is now a number of creams on the market that contain less than 10 milligrams an ounce, and these are unlikely to be effective.

Q: Why do you prefer creams instead of pills or capsules for progesterone?

A: Mother Nature guides us in this: The ovary never puts its hormones into the stomach, and for good reason. Progesterone is fat-soluble and, when absorbed from the stomach or intestines, it is taken by the portal vein directly to the liver, where it is efficiently metabolized for excretion in bile. When taken orally, about 85 to 90 percent of progesterone is lost via the bile or converted into metabolites that are not the same as real progesterone. Thus oral doses must be 100 to 200 milligrams per day, 10 to 20 times greater than transdermal doses, just to get the 20 to 24 milligrams needed daily. I see no reason to put the liver to all this work just to get 10 to 15 percent of the progesterone into the blood stream.

Natural progesterone is well absorbed through the skin into the fat layer under the skin and then into the bloodstream, riding on fatty components such as chylomicrons and red blood cell membranes. (Being fat-soluble, very little of the skin-absorbed progesterone is found in the watery blood serum.) Most of the good progesterone creams provide 480 milligrams of progesterone per ounce. If used up over 24 days in a month, one ounce provides 20 milligrams a day, the same daily amount usually made by an ovulating ovary. Our goal is to achieve equivalence with normal physiologic progesterone levels. Transdermal progesterone does this easily. There is no need to take oral doses of 100 to 200 milligrams per day.

Q: How can I check my hormone levels?

A: In the past, blood serum levels were used. However, the newer saliva hormone assays are probably better. When the ovaries make estrogen and progesterone for circulation in the watery blood serum, they bind them to protein (sex hormone–binding globulin in the case of estrogen or cortisol-binding globulin in the case of progesterone) to make them more water-soluble. Protein-bound hormones are not biologically active, but they represent over 90 percent of the hormones found in the serum. Thus the serum results do not accurately reflect the biologically available hormones.

Saliva hormones reflect only the biologically available hormones. Saliva hormone assays are less expensive, very accurate, easier to obtain, and more relevant than serum assays.

Since progesterone levels are apt to be highest two or three days after ovulation, it is wise to check hormone levels around day 18 to 21 of the menstrual month, counting day one as the first day of the preceding period. If the levels are found to be low at that time, you can be sure you are missing ovulation that month and your body progesterone level will be low.

(See the Resources section on page 334 for more information.)

Q: Can I use progesterone for birth control?

A: Folklore describes herbal and other plant sources (including Mexican wild yam) as being effective for birth control. Theoretically, progesterone or progestational effects are the key mechanism since, if taken early in the cycle, they could inhibit ovulation as the progestins in birth control pills do. However, I have no clinical experience using natural progesterone for this purpose and am unaware of any scientific studies testing this hypothesis, and therefore cannot recommend it.

GLOSSARY

amenorrhea	absence of menstruation
androgenic	producing masculine characteristics
anovulatory	suspension or cessation of ovulation
carcinogen	any cancer-producing substance
catalyst	any substance that enhances the rate or velocity of a chemical reaction
chromosome	a molecule that comprises the gene (genome), or hereditary factor, composed of DNA or RNA
conjugated	in biochemistry, one compound combined with another
corpus luteum	small yellow glandular mass in the ovary formed by an ovarian follicle after ovulation (release of its egg [ovum])
corticosteroid	hormone produced by the adrenal cortex
cytoplasm	the watery protoplasm of a cell, excluding the nucleus
diuretic	substance that increases urine production
DNA	deoxyribonucleic acid, the basic molecular subunit of chromosomes
dysmenorrhea	painful menstruation
endocrine	refers to organs (glands) that secrete hormones

327

endogenous	developing or originating within the body
endometrium	the inner lining of the uterus
enzyme	an organic compound, usually a protein, capable of facilitating a specific chemical reaction
exogenous	originating outside of the body
follicle	a very small sac or cavity composed of cells, e.g., the ovarian follicle that produces the ovum
gonadal	refers to the gamete-producing glands, i.e., ovaries and testes
gonadotropic	refers to hormones that affect or stimulate gonads
gram	unit of mass (weight); about one-twenty-eighth of an ounce
homeostasis	the body's ability to maintain a stable internal environment
hydroxylation	the addition of a hydroxyl radical (-OH) to a compound
hypermenorrhea	excessive bleeding with menses
hypothalamus	neural centers of the limbic brain just above the pituitary that control visceral activities, water balance, sleep, and hormone production by the pituitary
hysterectomy	surgical removal of the uterus
libido	sex drive
limbic brain	brain cortex below the corpus callosum and above the pituitary that contains neural centers controlling autonomic functions, homeostasis, and emotional sensation and responses, and regulates immune responses
luteinizing	refers to the maturation of ovarian follicles following ovulation, during which the follicle become the corpus luteum producing progesterone
mastodynia	painful breasts

metabolism	the biochemical process of living organisms by which substances are produced and energy is made available to the organism
microgram	one-millionth (10^{-6}) of a gram
milligram	one-thousandth (10^{-3}) of a gram
mineralcorticoid	an adrenal hormone that regulates sodium, potassium, and water balance
mitochondria	small organelles within the cytoplasm that are the site of converting sugar into energy
nanogram	one-billionth (10^{-9}) of a gram
oocyte	the cell that produces the ovum
oophorectomy	surgical removal of an ovary or ovaries
osteoblast	bone cell that forms new bone
osteoclast	bone cell that resorbs old bone
osteocyte	means bone cell; may become an osteoclast or an osteoblast
osteoid	the noncellular, collagenous matrix of bone
peptide	a class of low-molecular-weight compounds composed of several amino acids; a miniprotein
perimenopausal	referred to as premenopausal in this book—refers to the time preceding menopause when hormone changes are occurring
phyto-	denotes relationship to plants
premenopausal	prior to menopause, also called "perimenopausal"
resorption	the loss or dissolving away of a substance
serum	the watery, noncellular liquid of the blood
steroid	group name for compounds based on the cholesterol molecule, e.g., sex hormones and corticosteroids
sterol	compounds with a single hydroxyl group (-OH) soluble in fats, widely found in plants and animals. Cholesterol is a sterol.

synovial	referring to the inner lining of a joint
thermogenic	capable of inducing a rise in temperature
trans-	prefix referring to something altered from the natural state, such as transfatty acids
xeno-	combining form meaning strange or foreign

RECOMMENDED READING

Austin, Steve, N.D., and Cathy Hitchcock, M.S.W. *Breast Cancer: What You Should Know (But May Not Be Told) About Prevention, Diagnosis, and Treatment.* Rocklin, CA 95677: Prima Publishing, P.O. Box 1260BK, 1992.

Barnard, Neal, M.D. *Eat Right, Live Longer.* New York: Harmony Books, 1995.

Boston Women's Health Collective. *The New Our Bodies, Ourselves.* New York: Simon & Schuster, 1992.

Brown, Ellen, and Lynne Walker. *Breezing Through the Change.* Berkeley, CA: Frog, Ltd., P.O. Box 12327, 1994.

Coney, Sandra. *The Menopause Industry: How the Medical Establishment Exploits Women.* Alameda, CA: Hunter House, 1994.

DeMarco, Carolyn, M.D. *Take Charge of Your Body.* Winlaw, BC, VOG 2JO, Canada: The Well Woman Press, P.O. Box 66, 1994.

Ford, Gillian. *What's Wrong with My Hormones?* Newcastle, CA 95658: Desmond Ford Publications, 7955 Bullard Drive, 1992.

Gaby, Alan R., M.D. *Preventing and Reversing Osteoporosis.* Rocklin, CA 95677: Prima Publishing, P.O. Box 1260BK, 1993.

Gittleman, Ann Louise. *Super Nutrition for Menopause.* New York: Pocket Books, 1993.

Greer, Germaine. *The Change: Women, Aging and Menopause.* New York: Fawcett Columbine, 1991.

Jefferies, William McK., M.D., F.A.C.P. *The Safe Uses of Cortisone.* Springfield, IL: Charles C Thomas Publisher, 1981.

Kamen, Betty. *Hormone Replacement Therapy: Yes or No?* Novato, CA 94948: Nutrition Encounter, Inc., P.O. Box 5847, 1993.

Kradjian, Robert. *Save Yourself from Breast Cancer.* New York: Berkley Books, 1994.

Lee, John R., M.D. *Natural Progesterone: The Multiple Roles of a Remarkable Hormone.* Sebastopol, CA 95473: BLL Publishing, P.O. Box 2068, 1995. ($12. This is my first, self-published book on progesterone, written for doctors and other health care professionals.)

Lopez, Andrew. *Natural Pest Control.* Malibu, CA 90265: The Invisible Gardener of Malibu, 29161 Heathercliff Road, Ste. 216-408, (800) 354-9296, 1994.

Mindell, Earl, R.Ph., Ph.D. *Earl Mindell's Soy Miracle.* New York: Simon & Schuster, 1995.

Murray, Michael, N.D., and Joseph Pizzorno, N.D. *Encyclopedia of Natural Medicine.* Rocklin, CA: Prima Publishing, 1991.

Neal, Kate. *Balancing Hormones Naturally.* London: ION Press, 1994.

Northrup, Christiane, M.D. *Women's Bodies, Women's Wisdom.* New York: Bantam Books, 1994.

Peat, Raymond. *Nutrition for Women.* Eugene, OR 97405: P.O. Box 5764, 1993.

———. *Progesterone in Orthomolecular Medicine.* 1993.

Rinzler, Carol Ann. *Estrogen and Breast Cancer: A Warning to Women.* New York: Macmillan Publishing, 1993.

Robbins, John. *Diet for a New America*. Walpole, NH 03608: Stillpoint Publishing, Box 640, 1987.

————. *Diet for a New World*. New York: Avon Books, 1992. (Robbins has a new book coming out. I've read a chapter and it's excellent.)

Steinman, David. *Diet for a Poisoned Planet: How to Choose Safe Foods for You and Your Family*. New York: Ballantine Books, 1990. (Steinman has a new book coming out on pesticides, which I'm sure will be excellent.)

Stewart, Felicia, M.D., Felicia Guest, Gary Stewart, M.D., and Robert Hatcher, M.D. *My Body, My Health: The Concerned Woman's Guide to Gynecology*. New York: John Wiley & Sons, 1979.

West, Stanley, M.D. *The Hysterectomy Hoax*. New York: Doubleday, 1994.

RESOURCES

Sources of Natural Progesterone Supplements

Kenogen, P.O. Box 5764, Eugene, OR 97440-0564. (503) 345-9855. This is Ray Peat's progesterone in vitamin E oil, called Pro-gest-E Complex.

Professional & Technical Services, Inc., 621 S.W. Alder, Suite 900, Portland, OR 97205-3627. (503) 226-1010. Toll-free (800) 888-6814 (regular customers) and (800) 866-9085 (professionals). Fax (503) 226-6455.

Women's International Pharmacy, 5708 Monona Drive, Madison, WI 53716-3152. (608) 221-7800. Toll-free (800) 279-5708.

Health Watchers Systems, 13402 N. Scottsdale Rd., Suite B 150, Scottsdale, AZ 85254. (800) 321-6917.

Karuna Corporation, 42 Digital Drive, Suite 7, Novato, CA. 94949. (800) 826-7225.

Sources of Salivary Hormone Tests

Aeron Lab
1933 Davis St., Suite 310
San Leandro, CA 94577
(800) 631-7900
fax (510) 729-0383

334

Diagnos-Techs, Inc.
6620 192nd Place, Suite J-104
Kent, WA 98032
(800) 878-3787
(206) 251-0637

Recommended Alternative Health Newsletters

Alternatives (Dr. David G. Williams). One year, 12 issues, $69. Mountain Home Publishing, 2700 Cummings Lane, Kerrville, TX 78028, or call (210) 367-4492.

The Mindell Letter (Dr. Earl Mindell and Virginia Hopkins). One year, 12 issues, $69. Philips Publishing Inc., 7811 Montrose Rd., Potomac, MD 20854, or call (800) 787-3003.

Nutrition and Healing (Drs. Alan Gaby and Jonathan Wright). One year, 12 issues, $49. Publishers Mgt. Corp., P.O. Box 84909, Phoenix, AZ 85071, or call (800) 528-0559.

REFERENCES

Chapter 1

Reference texts used in this chapter:

Goodman, Louis S., and Alfred Gilman. *The Pharmacological Basis of Therapeutics*, 8th edition. Toronto: The Macmillan Company, 1990: chapter 58.

Textbook of Clinical Chemistry. Norbert W. Tietz, Ph.D., ed. Philadelphia: W.B. Saunders Co., 1986:1085–1171.

Thomas, J. Hywel, and Brian Gillham. *Will's Biochemical Basis of Medicine*. 2d edition. Oxford: Butterworth-Heinemann Ltd., 1989: chapter 17.

Chapter 2

Morley, John E., M.B., 1994. Nutritional modulation of behavior and immunocompetence. *Nutrition Reviews* August, 52(8):S6–S8.

Reference texts used in this chapter:

Goodman, Louis S., and Alfred Gilman. *The Pharmacological Basis of Therapeutics*. 8th edition. Toronto: The Macmillan Company, 1990: chapter 58.

Textbook of Clinical Chemistry. Norbert W. Tietz, Ph.D., ed. Philadelphia: W.B. Saunders Co., 1986:1085–1171.

Will's Biochemical Basis of Medicine. 2d edition. Oxford: Butterworth-Heinemann Ltd., 1989: chapter 17.

Chapter 3

Rinzler, Carol Ann. *Estrogen and Breast Cancer.* New York: Macmillan Publishing Co., 1993:31–32.

Strauss, S. 1988. A capsulated history of drug law in the U.S. *U.S. Pharmacist.* November.

Seaman, Barbara, and Gideon Seaman. *Women and the Crisis in Sex Hormones.* New York: Rawson Associates, 1977:82.

Vaughn, Paul. *The Pill on Trial.* London: Weidenfeld and Nicolson, 1970:25.

Coney, Sandra. *The Menopause Industry.* Alameda, CA: Hunter House, 1994.

References for Prior article, "One Voice on Menopause"

Prior, J. C. "One Voice on Menopause," *JAMWA* 49, no. 1 (January/February 1994):27–29.

Prior, J. C., B. Ho Yuen, P. Clement, et al. 1992. Reversible luteal phase changes and infertility associated with marathon training. *Lancet* 1:269–70.

Prior, J. C., and Y. M. Vigna. 1991. Ovulation disturbances and exercise training. *Clin Obstet Gynecol* 26:180–90.

Prior, J. C., Y. M. Vigna, N. Alojado, et al. 1987. Conditioning exercise decreases premenstrual symptoms: a prospective controlled six-month trial. *FertilSteril* 47:402–406.

Prior, J. C., Y. M. Vigna, M. T. Schechter, and A. E. Burgess. 1990. Spinal bone loss and ovulatory disturbances. *New England Journal of Medicine* 323:1221–27.

Sherman, B. M., J. H. West, and S. G. Korenmam. 1976. The menopausal transition: analysis of LH, FSH, estradiol and progesterone concentrations during menstrual cycles of older women. *J Clin Endocrinol Metab* 42:629–36.

Albright, F. 1936. Studies in ovarian function III: the menopause. *Endocrinology* 20:24.

Reyes, F. L., J. S. Winter, and C. Paiman. 1977. Pituitary ovarian relationships preceding the menopause: a cross-sectional study of serum follicle-stimulating hormone, luteinizing hormone, prolactin, estradiol and progesterone levels. *American Journal of Obstetrics and Gynecology* 129:557–64.

Tilt, E. J. *The Change of Life in Health and Disease. A Practical Treatise on the Nervous and Other Affections Incidental to Women at the Decline of Life.* Philadelphia: Lindsay and Blakiston, 1871.

Jaszman, I, N. D. Van Lith, and J. C. Saat. 1969. The perimenopausal symptoms: the statistical analysis of a survey. Parts A and B. *Medical Gynecology Sociology* 4:268–76.

Kaufert, P. A., P. Gilbert, and R. Tate. 1987. Defining menopausal status: the impact of longitudinal data. *Maturitas* 9:217–26.

Neugarten, B. L., and R. J. Kraines. 1964. Menopausal symptoms in women of various ages. *Psychom Med* 27:266–73.

Leather, A. T., M. Savras, and J. W. Stuidd. 1991. Endometrial histology and bleeding patterns after eight years of continuous combined estrogen and progestin therapy in postmenopausal women. *Obstet Gynecol* 78:1008–10.

Gallagher, J. C., W. T. Kable, and D. Goldgar. 1991. The effect of progestin therapy on cortical and trabecular bone: comparison with estrogen. *American Journal of Medicine* 90:171–78.

Jayo, M. J., D. S. Weaver, M. R. Adams, and S. E. Rankin. 1990. Effects on bone of surgical menopause and estrogen therapy with or without progesterone replacement in cynomolgus monkeys. *American Journal of Obstetrics and Gynecology* 614:618.

Prior, J. C. 1990. Progesterone as a bone-trophic hormone. *Endocr Rev* 11:386–98.

―――. 1991. Postmenopausal estrogen therapy and cardiovascular disease (letter). *New England Journal of Medicine* 326:705–706.

Barret-Conner, E. 1991. Postmenopausal estrogen and prevention bias. *Annals of Internal Medicine* 115:455–56.

Coronary Drug Project Research Group. 1973. Coronary drug project: findings leading to the discontinuation of the 2.5 mg/day estrogen group. *Journal of the American Medical Association* (hereafter cited as *JAMA*) 226:652–57.

―――. 1978. Coronary drug project: estrogens and cancer (letter). *JAMA* 239:2758–59.

Byyny, R. L., and L. Speroff. *A Clinical Guide for the Care of Older Women.* Baltimore: Williams & Wilkins, 1990.

McKinlay, S. M., D. J. Brambilla, and J. G. Posner. 1992. The normal menopausal transition. *Maturitas* 14:103–15.

Chapter 4

Ellison, P. T., C. Panter-Brick, S. F. Lipson, and M. T. O'Rourke. 1993. The ecological context of human ovarian function. *Human Reproduction* 8:2248–58.

Raloff, J. 1993. Ecocancers. *Science News,* July 3, 144:10–13 and reported in article Sperm-count drop tied to pollution rise. *Medical Tribune,* March 26, 1992.

Documenta Geigy. *Scientific Tables.* 6th edition. Ardsley, NY: Geigy Pharmaceuticals: 493.

Lennon, H. M., H. H. Wotiz, L. Parsons, and P. J. Mozden. 1966. Reduced estriol excretion in patients with breast cancer prior to endocrine therapy. *JAMA* 196:112–20.

Raz, R., and W. E. Stamm. 1993. A controlled trial of intravaginal estriol in postmenopausal women with recurrent urinary tract infections. *New England Journal of Medicine* 329: 753–56.

Campbell, B. C., and P. T. Ellison. 1992. Menstrual variation in salivary testosterone among regularly cycling women. *Horm Res* 37:132–36.

Rose, D. P. *Obstets & Gynecol,* 1977.

Lipsett, M. P. Steroid hormones, in *Reproductive Endocrinology, Physiology, and Clinical Management.* Yen, S.S.C., and R. B. Jaffe, eds. Philadelphia: W. B. Saunders Co., 1978: 80.

Human Reproduction, December 1993.

Chapter 5

McLachlan, John, diagram "Hormonal mimic" taken from 1993. Functional toxicology: a new approach to detect biologically active xenobiotics, published in *Environmental Health Perspectives* 10:386–87.

Hileman, Beth. 1994. Reproductive estrogens linked to reproductive abnormalities, cancer. *Chemical and Engineering News,* January 31: 19–23.

Lemonick, Michael D. 1994. Not so fertile ground. *Time,* September 19: 68–70.

Weiss, Rick. 1994. Estrogen in the environment. *The Washington Post,* January 25: 10–13.

Raloff, J. 1993. Ecocancers. *Science News* 144, July 3: 10–13.

———. 1994. The gender benders. *Science News* 145, January 8: 24–27.

———. 1994. That feminine touch. *Science News* 145, January 22: 56–59.

Cone, Marla. 1994. Sexual confusion in the wild. Pollution's effect on sexual development fires debate. Battle looms on chemicals that disrupt hormones. 3-part series. *The Los Angeles Times,* October 2–4.

Begley, S., and D. Glick. 1994. The estrogen complex. *Newsweek,* March 21: 76–77.

Colborn, T., F. S. vom Saal, and A. M. Soto. 1993. Developmental effects of endocrine-disrupting chemicals in wildlife and humans. *Environmental Health Perspectives* 10:378–84.

Chapter 6

History of progesterone as described by Goodman & Gilman. *The Pharmacological Basis of Therapeutics.* 6th edition, 1980: chapter 61 (Estrogens and Progestins: 1420), and *Textbook of Clinical Chemistry.* Norbert W. Tietz, Ph.D., ed. Philadelphia: W.B. Saunders Co., 1986: 1085–1171.

Elks, M. L. 1993. Peripheral effects of sex steroids: implications for patient management. *JAMWA* 48:41–45.

Roof, Robin, et al. of Rutgers University. 1993. Reported in *The Economist,* December 11, 329:35.

Stampfer, M. J., G. A. Colditz, W. C. Willett, et al. 1991. Postmenopausal estrogen therapy and cardiovascular disease—ten-year follow-up from the Nurses' Questionnaire Study. *New England Journal of Medicine* 325:756–62.

Witt, D. M., L. J. Young, and D. Crews. 1994. Progesterone and sexual behavior in males. *Psychoneuroendocrinology* 19:553–56.

DeBold, J. F., and C. A. Frye. 1994. Progesterone and the neural mechanisms of hamster sexual behavior. *Psychoneuroendocrinology* 19:563–66.

Campbell, B. C., and P. T. Ellison. 1992. Menstrual variation in salivary testosterone among regularly cycling women. *Horm Res* 37:132–36.

Swerdloff, R. S., and C. Wang. 1993. Androgen deficiency and aging in men. *WJM* 159:579–84.

Reference texts used in this chapter:

Goodman, Louis S., and Alfred Gilman. *The Pharmacological Basis of Therapeutics.* 8th edition. Toronto: The Macmillan Company, 1990: chapter 58.

Textbook of Clinical Chemistry. Norbert W. Tietz, Ph.D., ed. Philadelphia: W. B. Saunders Co., 1986: 1085–1171.

Thomas, J. Hywel, and Brian Gillham. *Will's Biochemical Basis of Medicine.* 2d edition. Oxford: Butterworth-Heinemann Ltd., 1989: chapter 17.

Chapter 7

Hargrove, J. T., W. S. Maxson, A. C. Wentz, and L. S. Burnett. 1989. Menopausal hormone replacement therapy with continuous daily oral micronized estradiol and progesterone. *Obstetrics & Gynecology* 71:606–12.

The Writing Group for the PEPI Trial, 1995. Effects of estrogen or estrogen/progestin regimens on heart disease risk factors in postmenopausal women: The postmenopausal estrogen/progestins interventions (PEPI) trial. *JAMA,* January 18. 273(3):240–41.

Whitehead, M. I., D. Fraser, L. Schenkel, D. Crook, and J. C. Stevenson. 1990. Transdermal administration of oestrogen/progestagen hormone replacement therapy. *Lancet* 335:310–12.

Stevenson, J. C., K. F. Ganger, et al. 1990. Effects of transdermal versus oral hormone replacement therapy on bone density in spine and proximal femur in postmenopausal women. *Lancet* 336:265-26.

Crane, M. G., and J. J. Harris. Effects of gonadal hormones on plasma renin activity and aldosterone excretion rate, in *Meta-*

bolic *Effects of Gonadal Hormones and Contraceptive Steroids.* H. A. Salhanick, D. M. Kipnis, and R. L. Vande Weile, eds. New York: Plenum Press, 1969: 446–46, and discussion: 736.

Crane, M. G., J. J. Harris, and W. Winsor III. 1971. Hypertension, oral contraceptive agents, and conjugated estrogens. *Annals of Internal Medicine* 74:13–21.

Landau, R. L., and K. Lugibihl. 1961. The catabolic and natriuretic effects of progesterone in man. *Recent Progress in Hormone Research.* 17:249–81.

Edgren, R. A. Progestagens. Reprinted from *Clinical Use of Sex Steroids.* Chicago: Year Book Medical Publishers, Inc., 1980.

Ottoson, U. B., B. G. Johansson, and B. von Schoultz. 1985. Subfractions of high-density lipoprotein cholesterol during estrogen replacement therapy: a comparison between progestogens and natural progesterone. *American Journal of Obstetrics and Gynecology* 151:746–50.

1995. The writing group for the PEPI trial. *JAMA* 273:199–208.

Gambrell, R. D. 1982. The menopause: benefits and risks of estrogen-progestogen replacement therapy. *Fertil Steril* 37: 457–74.

1989. *Medical Times* Sept: 35–43.

Scientific American Medicine, updated 1992. New York: *Scientific American*, chapter 15 (X):9.

Bergkvist, L., H.-O. Adami, I. Persson, R. Hoover, and C. Schairer. 1989. The risk of breast cancer after estrogen and estrogen-progestin replacement. *New England Journal of Medicine* 321: 293–97.

Chapter 8

Leary, Warren E. 1995. Progesterone may play major role in the prevention of nerve disease. *New York Times*, June 27, C3.

Roof, R. L., et al. 1993. Gender influences outcome of brain injury: progesterone plays a protective role. *Brain Res.*, April 2, 607(1-2):333–36.

————. 1994. Progesterone facilitates cognitive recovery and reduces secondary neuronal loss caused by cortical contusion injury in male rats. *Exp Neurol*, September, 129(1):64–69.

Harris, Brian. 1994. Maternity blues and major endocrine changes: Cardiff puerperal mood and hormone study II, Wales. *British Medical Journal*, April 19, 308:949–53.

Braverman, Eric. 1993. New era in hormone therapy. *Total Health* 7, no. 4 (August): 31.

————. 1991. Natural estrogen and progesterone research indicates health benefits of natural vs. synthetic hormones. *Total Health* 13, no. 5 (October): 55.

Chapter 9

Kaplan, Abraham, M.D. *The Nervous System*, Volume I, the Hypothalamus Supplement. Illustrated by Frank H. Netter, M. D. New York: CIBA, 1957:147–65. (A good presentation of the functions and neural systems of the limbic brain.)

Prior, J. C., Y. M. Vigna, M. T. Schechter, et al. 1990. Spinal bone loss and ovulatory disturbances. *New England Journal of Medicine* 323:1221–27.

Campbell, B. C., and P. T. Ellison. 1992. Menstrual variation in salivary testosterone among regularly cycling women. *Horm Res* 37:132–36.

Stevenson, J. C., K. F. Ganger, et al. 1990. Effects of transdermal versus oral hormone replacement therapy on bone density in spine and proximal femur in postmenopausal women. *Lancet* 336:265–69.

Chapter 10

Belchetz, P. E. 1994. Hormonal treatment of postmenopausal women. *New England Journal of Medicine* 330:1062–71.

Velde, E. R. 1993. Disappearing ovarian follicles and reproductive aging (letter). *Lancet* 341: 1125.

Leridon, H. *Human Fertility: The Basic Components.* Chicago: University of Chicago Press, 1977:202.

Van Noord-Zaadstra, B. M., C.W.N. Looman, H. Alsback, et al. 1991. Delaying childbearing: effect of age on fecundity and outcome of pregnancy. *British Medical Journal* 302: 1361–65.

Lees, B., T. Molleson, T. R. Arnett, and J. C. Stevenson. 1993. Differences in proximal femur bone density over two centuries. *Lancet* 341:673–75.

Textbook of Clinical Chemistry. Philadelphia: W. B. Saunders Co., 1986: 1088.

Chapter 11

Prior, J. C., and Y. M. Vigna. 1990. Spinal bone loss and ovulatory disturbances. *New England Journal of Medicine* 223:1221–27.

Prior, J. C., Y. M. Vigna, and N. Alojado. 1991. Progesterone and the prevention of osteoporosis, *Canadian Journal of Obstetrics/Gynecology & Women's Health Care* 3:178–84.

Prior, J. C. 1990. Progesterone as a bone-trophic hormone. *Endocrine Reviews* 11:386–98.

Ebeling, P., and V. A. Koivisto. 1994. Physiological importance of dehydroepiandrosterone. *Lancet* 343:147981.

The Biologic Role of Dehydroepiandrosterone. M. Kalimi and W. Regelson, ed. Walter de Gruyter, 1990.

Ebeling, P., and V. A. Koivisto. 1994. Physiological importance of dehydroepiandrosterone. *Lancet* 343:147981.

Chapter 12

Albright, F., P. H. Smith, and A. M. Richardson. 1941. Post-menopausal osteoporosis: its clinical features. *JAMA* 116:2465–74.

Aitken, M., D. M. Hart, and R. Lindsay. 1973. Oestrogen replacement therapy for prevention of osteoporosis after oopherectomy. *British Medical Journal* 3:515–18.

Coats, C. 1990. Negative effects of a high-protein diet. *Family Practice Recertification* 12:80-88.

Lindsay, R., D. M. Hart, C. Forrest, and C. Baird. 1980. Prevention of spinal osteoporosis in oophorectomized women. *Lancet* II:1151–54.

Gordon, G. S., J. Picchi, and B. S. Root. 1973. Antifracture efficacy of long-term estrogens for osteoporosis. *Trans Assoc Am Physicians* 86:326–32.

Hammond, C. B., F. R. Jelvsek, K. L. Lee, W. T. Creasman, and R. T. Parker. 1979. Effects of long-term estrogen replacement therapy. I. Metabolic effects. *American Journal of Obstetrics and Gynecology* 133:525–36.

Hutchinson, T. A., S. M. Polansky, and A. R. Feinstein. 1979. Postmenopausal oestrogens protect against fractures of hip and distal radius: a case control study. *Lancet* II: 705–709.

Weiss, N. S., C. L. Ure, J. H. Ballard, A. R. Williams, and J. R. Daling. 1980. Decreased risk of fracture of hip and lower forearm with postmenopausal use of estrogen. *New England Journal of Medicine* 303:1195–98.

Ettinger, B., H. K. Genant, and C. E. Cann. 1985. Long-term estrogen replacement therapy prevents bone loss and fractures. *Annals of Internal Medicine* 102:319–24.

Barzel, U. S. 1988. Estrogens in the prevention and treatment of postmenopausal osteo-porosis: a review. *American Journal of Medicine* 85:847–50.

Christiansen, C., M. S. Christiansen, and I. Transbol. 1981. Bone mass in postmenopausal women after withdrawal of oestrogen/progestagen replacement therapy. *Lancet* February 28: 459–61.

Manolagas, S. C., R. L. Jilka, G. Hangoc, et al. 1992. Increased osteoclast development after estrogen loss: mediation by interleukin-6. *Science* 257:88–91.

Felson, D. T., Y. Zhang, M. T. Hannan, D. P. Kiel, P.W.F. Wilson, and J. J. Anderson. 1993. The effect of postmenopausal estrogen therapy on bone density in elderly women. *New England Journal of Medicine* 329:1141–46.

Ellison, P. T., C. Panter-Brick, S. F. Lipson, and M. T. O'Rourke. 1993. The ecological context of human ovarian function. *Human Reproduction* 8:2248–58.

Prior, J. C., and V. M. Vigna. 1990. Spinal bone loss and ovulatory disturbances. *New England Journal of Medicine* 323:1221–27.

Rudy, D. R. 1990. Hormone replacement therapy. *Postgraduate Medicine* December: 157–64.

Cummings, S. R., M. C. Nevitt, W. S. Browner, et al. 1995. Risk factors for hip fracture in white women. *New England Journal of Medicine* 332:767–73.

Riggs, B. L., H. W. Wahner, L. J. Melton., et al. 1986. Rates of bone loss in the appendicular and axial skeleton of women: evidence of substantial vertebral bone loss before menopause. *J Clin Invest* 77:1487–91.

Prior, J. C., Y. M. Vigna, and N. Alojado. 1991. Progesterone and the prevention of osteoporosis. *Canadian Journal of Obstetrics/Gynecology & Women's Health Care* 3:178–84.

Prior, J. C. 1990. Progesterone as a bone-trophic hormone. *Endocrine Reviews* 11: 386–98.

Prior, J. C., Y. M. Vigna, and R. Burgess. Medroxyprogesterone acetate increases trabecular bone density in women with menstrual disorder. Presented at the annual meeting of the Endocrine Society, Indianapolis, June 11, 1987.

Munk-Jensen, N., S. P. Nielsen, E. B. Obel, and P. B. Eriksen. 1988. Reversal of postmenopausal vertebral bone loss by oestrogen and progestagen: a double-blind placebo-controlled study. *British Medical Journal* 296:1150–52.

Johansen, J. S., S. B. Jensen, B. J. Riis, et al. 1990. Bone formation is stimulated by combined estrogen, progestagen. *Metabolism* 39:1122–26.

Cundy, T., M. Evans, H. Roberts, et al. 1991. Bone density in women receiving a depot medroxyprogesterone acetate for contraception. *British Medical Journal* 303:13–16.

Lee, J. R. 1990. Osteoporosis reversal: the role of progesterone. *Intern Clin Nutr Rev* 10:384–91.

———. 1990. Osteoporosis reversal with transdermal progesterone (letter). *Lancet* 336:1327.

———. 1991. Is natural progesterone the missing link in osteoporosis prevention and treatment? *Medical Hypotheses* 35:316–18.

Nolan, Charles R., M.D., et al. 1994. Aluminum and lead absorption from dietary sources in women ingesting calcium citrate. *Southern Medical Journal*. September, 87(9):894–98.

Lees, B., T. Molleson, T. R. Arnett, and J. C. Stevenson. 1993. Differences in proximal femur density over two centuries. *Lancet* 341:673–75.

Dalsky, G. P., K. S. Stocke, A. A. Ehsani, et al. 1988. Weight-bearing exercise training and femoral neck and lumbar spine bone mineral density. *Annals of Internal Medicine* 108:824–28.

Riggs, B. L., S. F. Hodgson, W. M. O'Fallon, E.Y.S. Chao, et al. 1990. Effect of fluoride treatment on the fracture rate in postmenopausal women with osteoporosis. *New England Journal of Medicine* 322:802–809.

Kleerekoper, M. E., E. Peterson, E. Phillips, D. Nelson, et al. 1989. Continuous sodium fluoride therapy does not reduce vertebral fracture rate in postmenopausal osteoporosis (abstract). *J Bone & Miner Res* 4 (Suppl. 1):S376.

Hedlund, L. R., and J. C. Gallagher. 1989. Increased incidence of hip fracture in osteoporotic women treated with sodium fluoride. *J Bone & Miner Res* 4:223–25.

Sowers, M.F.R., M. K. Clark, M. L. Jannausch, and R. B. Wallace. 1991. A prospective study of bone mineral content and fracture in communities with differential fluoride exposure. *American Journal of Epidemiology* 134:649–60.

Jacobsen, S. J., J. Goldberg, T. P. Miles, J. A. Brody, et al. 1990. Regional variation in the incidence of hip fractures: U.S. white women aged 65 years and older. *JAMA* 264:500–501.

Cooper, C., C.A.C. Wickham, D.J.R. Barker, and S. J. Jacobsen. 1991. Water fluoridation and hip fracture (letter). *JAMA* 266:513–14.

Danielson, C., J. L. Lyon, M. Egger, and G. K. Goodenough. 1992. Hip fractures and fluoridation in Utah's elderly population. *JAMA* 268:746–47.

Coats, C. 1990. Negative effects of a high-protein diet. *Family Practice Recertification* 12:80–88.

Chapter 13

Stampfer, M. J., G. A. Colditz, W. C. Willett, et al. 1991. Postmenopausal estrogen therapy and cardiovascular disease—10-

year follow-up from the Nurses' Questionnaire Study. *New England Journal of Medicine* 325:756–62.

Wilson, P.W.F., R. J. Garrison, and W. P. Castelli. 1985. Postmenopausal estrogen use, cigarette smoking, and cardiovascular morbidity in women over 50. *New England Journal of Medicine* 313: 1038–43.

Prior, J. C. 1992. Letter. *New England Journal of Medicine* 326: 705–706.

Tribble, D. L., and E. Frank. 1994. Dietary antioxidants, cancer, and atherosclerotic heart disease. *W J Med* 161:605–12.

Chapter 14

Somerville, Scott. *Connections*. Lewisville, TX: Life Dynamics, Inc., 1994. (To order this monograph, send $6.00 to Life Dynamics, Inc., P.O. Box 185, Lewisville, TX 75067)

Bergkvist, L., H.-O. Adami, I. Persson, R. Hoover, and C. Schairer. 1989. The risk of breast cancer after estrogen and estrogen-progestin replacement. *New England Journal of Medicine* 321:293–97.

Henderson, B. E., R. K. Ross, M. C. Pike, and J. T. Casagrande. 1982. Endogenous hormones as a major factor in human cancer. *Cancer Research* 42:3232–39.

Hoover, R., L. A. Gray, Sr., P. Cole, and B. MacMahon. 1976. Menopausal estrogens and breast cancer. *New England Journal of Medicine* 295:401–405.

Hiatt, R. A., R. Bawol, G. D. Friedman, and R. Hoover. 1984. Exogenous estrogen and breast cancer after bilateral oophorectomy. *Cancer* 54:139–44.

La Vecchia, C., A. Decarli, F. Parazzini, A. Gentile, C. Liberati, and S. Franceschi. 1986. Noncontraceptive oestrogens and the risk of breast cancer in women. *International Journal of Cancer* 38:853–58.

Astrow, Alan B., M.D. 1994. Rethinking cancer (letter). *Lancet* February 26.

Cowan, L. D., L. Gordis, J. A. Tonascia, and G. S. Jones. 1981. Breast cancer incidence in women with a history of progesterone deficiency. *American Journal of Epidemiology* 114:209–17.

Chang, K. J., et al. 1995. Influences of percutaneous administration of estradiol and progesterone on human breast epithelial cell cycle in vivo. *Fertility and Sterility* 63: 785–91.

A report by Ruby Senie, Ph.D., of the Centers for Disease Control, at the annual science writers seminar sponsored by the American Cancer Society. Reported by the February 5, 1992, issue of *Health* and by the May 7, 1992, issue of *Medical Tribune*.

Raloff, Janet. 1993. Ecocancers: do environmental factors underlie a breast cancer epidemic? *Science News,* July 3, 144:10–13.

Pike, M. C., D. V. Spicer, L. Dahmoush, and M. F. Press. 1993. Estrogens, progestogens, normal breast proliferation, and breast cancer risk. *Epidem Rev* 15:64–82.

Willett, W. C., M. J. Stampfer, M. B. Colditz, et al. 1987. Dietary fat and the risk of breast cancer. *New England Journal of Medicine* 316:22–28.

Ellison, P. T., C. Panter-Brick, S. F. Lipson, and M. T. O'Rourke. 1993. The ecological context of human ovarian function. *Human Reproduction* 8(12):2248–58.

Ellison, P. T. 1993. Measurements of salivary progesterone. *Annals of the New York Academy of Science* September 20, 694:161–76.

Ellison, P. T., S. F. Lipson, M. T. O'Rourke, et al. 1993. Population variation in ovarian function (letter). *Lancet* August 14, 342:433–34.

Campbell, B. C., and P. T. Ellison. 1992. Menstrual variation in salivary testosterone among regularly cycling women. *Horm Res* (Switzerland) 37:(4–5):132–36.

Kerlikowske, K., D. Grady, S. M. Rubin, et al. 1995. Efficacy of screening mammography. *JAMA* 273:149–54.

Miller, A. B., C. J. Baines, and T. Wall. 1992. Canadian national breast screening study 2: breast cancer detection and death rates among women aged 50 to 59 years. *Canadian Medical Association Journal* 147:1477–88.

Gruenigen, V. E., and J. R. Karlen. 1995. Carcinoma of the endometrium. *American Family Physician*, May 1: 1531–36.

Ellison, P. T., C. Panter-Brick, S. F. Lipson, and M. T. O'Rourke. 1993. The ecological context of human ovarian function. *Human Reproduction* 8:2248–58.

Scientific American Medicine, New York: *Scientific American,* 1992, updated, chapter 15 (X): 9.

Chapter 15

Jefferies, William, M.D. *The Safe Uses of Cortisone.* Springfield, IL: Charles C Thomas. Publisher, 1981.

Chapter 16

Crane, M. G., and J. J. Harris. Effects of gonadal hormones on plasma renin activity and aldosterone excretion rate. In H. A. Salhanick, D. M. Kipnis, and R. L. Vande Weile, eds. *Metabolic Effects of Gonadal Hormones and Contraceptive Steroids.* New York: Plenum Press, 1969: 446–63, and discussion: 736.

Crane, M. G., J. J. Harris, and W. Winsor III. 1971. Hypertension, oral contraceptive agents and conjugated estrogens. *Annals of Internal Medicine* 74:13–21.

Stampfer, M. J., G. A. Colditz, W. C. Willett, et al. 1991. Post-menopausal estrogen therapy and cardiovascular disease. *New England Journal of Medicine* 325:756–62.

Smith, E. P., J. Boyd, G. R. Frank, et al. 1994. Estrogen resistance caused by a mutation in the estrogen-receptor gene in a man. *New England Journal of Medicine* 331:1056–61.

Dalton, K. *The Premenstrual Syndrome and Progesterone Therapy.* Chicago: Year Book Medical Publishers, Inc., 1977.

DeBold, J. F., and C. A. Frye. 1994. Progesterone and the neural mechanisms of hamster sexual behavior. *Psychoneuroendocrinology* 19:563–79.

Witt, D. M., L. J. Young, and D. Crews. 1994. Progesterone and sexual behavior in males. *Psychoneuroendocrinology* 19:553–62.

1994. Maternity blues and major endocrine changes. *British Medical Journal*, April 9, 308:949–53.

Chapter 17

Melillo, Mark. 1994. Estrogen use may predispose women to lupus. *Medical Tribune*, November 17.

Chapter 18

Diaz-Zagoya, J. C., J. Laguna, and J. Guzman-Garcia. 1971. Studies on the regulation of cholesterol metabolism by the use of the structural analogue, diosgenin. *Biochem Pharmacol* 20(12): 3473–80.

Odumosu, A. 1982. How vitamin C, clofibrate and diosgenin control cholesterol metabolism in male guinea-pigs. *Int J Vitam Nutr Res* Suppl (Switzerland) 23: 187–95.

Juarez-Oropeza, M. A., J. C. Diaz-Zagoya, and J. L. Rabinowitz.

1987. In vivo and in vitro studies of hypocholesterolemic effects of diosgenin in rats. *International Journal of Biochemistry* 19 (8): 679–83.

Chapter 19

Erasmus, Udo. *Fats that Heal, Fats that Kill*. Burnaby, BC, Canada: Alive Books, 1993.

Willett, W. C., M. J. Stampfer, G. A. Colditz, F. E. Speizer, et al. 1993. Intake of trans fatty acids and risk of coronary heart disease among women. *Lancet* 341:581–85.

Laino, C. 1994. Trans-fatty acids in margarine can increase MI risk. *Circulation*, 89:94–101.

Trichopoulous, Antonia, M.D., et al. 1995. Consumption of olive oil and specific food groups in relation to breast cancer risk in Greece. *Journal of the National Cancer Institute*, January 18, 87(2):110–16.

1994. Foods that may prevent breast cancer: studies are investigating soybeans, whole wheat and green tea among others. *Primary Care and Cancer* 14(2):10–11.

Toniolo, Paolo, et al. 1994. Consumption of meat, animal products, protein and fat and risk of breast cancer: a prospective cohort study in New York. *Epidemiology*, July, 5(4):391–96.

1994. Dietary changes in arthritis. *The Practitioner*, June, 238:443–48.

Semplicini, Andrea and Valle. 1994. Fish oils and their possible role in the treatment of cardiovascular diseases. *Pharmac Ther* 61:385–97.

Schmidt, Erik Berg, and Jorn Dyerberg. 1994. Omega-3 fatty acids—current status in cardiovascular medicine. *Drugs* 47(3):405–24.

Rogers, Adrianne E., et al. 1993. Diet and carcinogenesis. *Carcinogenesis* 14(11):2205–17.

Miller, A. B., et al. 1994. Diet in the etiology of cancer: a review. *European Journal of Cancer* 30A(2):207–28.

Austoker, Joan. 1994. Diet and cancer. *British Medical Journal* 308:1610–14.

The Biologic Role of Dehydroepiandrosterone. M. Kalimi and W. Regelson, ed. Walter de Gruyter, 1990.

Diaz-Zagoya, J. C., J. Laguna, and J. Guzman-Garcia. 1971. Studies on the regulation of cholesterol metabolism by the use of the structural analogue, diosgenin. *Biochem Pharmacol* 20(12): 3473–80.

Odumosu, A. 1982. How vitamin C, clofibrate and diosgenin control cholesterol metabolism in male guinea-pigs. *Int J Vitam Nutr Res* Suppl (Switzerland) 23: 187–95.

Juarez-Oropeza, M. A., J. C. Diaz-Zagoya, and J. L. Rabinowitz. 1987. In vivo and in vitro studies of hypocholesterolemic effects of diosgenin in rats. *International Journal of Biochemistry* 19 (8): 679–83.

Schell, O. *Modern Meat.* New York: Vintage Books, Random House, 1985: 283–84 and 287.

Blaylock, Russell L., M.D. *Excitotoxins: The Taste that Kills.* Santa Fe: Health Press, 1994.

Chapter 20

Verschuren, Monique W. M., et al. 1995. Serum total cholesterol and long-term coronary heart disease mortality in different cultures. *JAMA*, July 12, 274 (2).

APPENDIX: THE STRUCTURE OF STEROID HORMONES

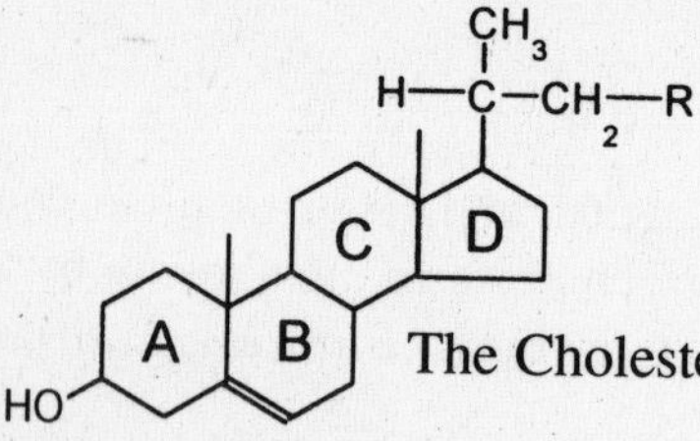

The Cholesterol Molecule

Figure 18: Notice the four rings, labeled A, B, C, and D, that make up the main chassis of the molecule. These are the four rings that characterize all the steroid hormones. In the following figure are three such hormones.

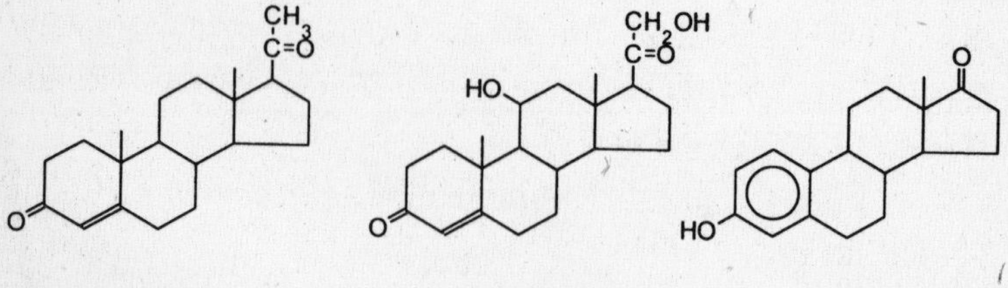

progesterone   corticosterone   estrone

Figure 19: Notice how the basic structure of cholesterol, the precursor to the steroid hormones, remains the same in three different steroid hormones. Slight molecular variations produce hormones that create enormous variations in humans.

Note that all of these steroid hormones retain the similar four-ring structure of the cholesterol molecule. They differ, however, in the atoms attached at various places to the basic structure. The differences appear minor, though their actions are thereby changed considerably. Others, like estrone (and all estrogens), have a different A-ring. This ring, depicted with a circle inside, indicates it has had three hydrogens removed, leaving three sets of double bonds circulating around the ring of carbon atoms making up the six-sided ring. This is what chemists call a benzene ring. However, with the presence of the -OH group at the side of the ring farthest away from the rest of the molecule, this ring is called a phenol ring. Among the steroid hormones, only estrogen molecules have a phenol ring. Nearly all of the xenoestrogens have phenol rings.

The body does not build these various important steroid hormones on different assembly lines. Cholesterol is the main building block. Tiny energy packets (mitochondria) within each and every cell of the body can substitute and rearrange some atoms at the top of cholesterol's D-ring, creating a new version called pregnenolone. As it passes through the bloodstream to the ovaries and adrenal glands, pregnenolone can then be transformed into progesterone or (almost identical) 17-OH-pregnenolone. Then, from these two steroids, all the other steroid hormones can be made by relatively minor molecular modifications, depending on body need. In this sort of production, one steroid is transformed into another. Many of the intermediate steps in this pathway are active hormones in their own right, even though they also serve by being transformed into still other hormones. At the end of the transformational paths are aldosterone, cortisol, and the estrogens, which are fated to be metabolized and excreted from the body.

Although the steroid hormones are remarkably similar in shape, each of them has markedly different effects, and these differences arise from very slight variations in their molecular structure.

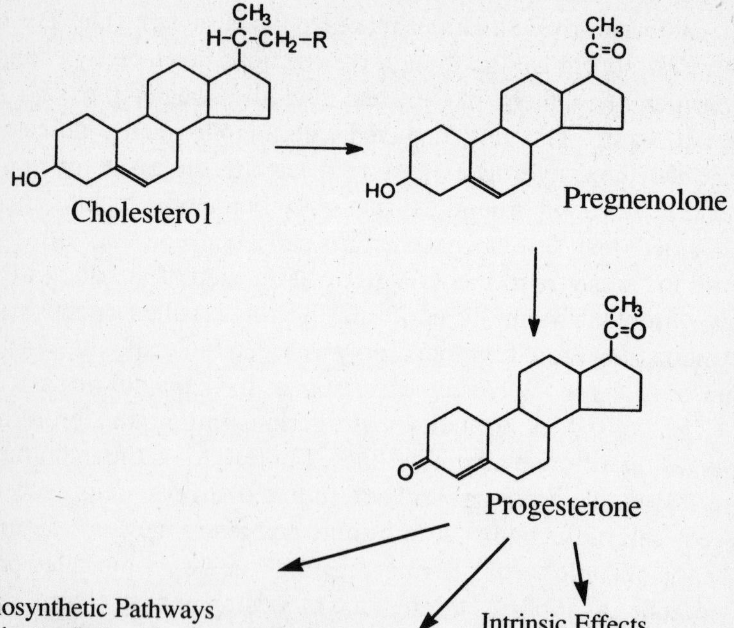

Biosynthetic Pathways
androstenedione
testosterone
estrone, estradiol, estriol
all cortisol and
    corticosteroids
aldosterone

Reproductive Effects
secretory endometrium
survival of embryo
development of fetus
    throughout gestation
libido

Intrinsic Effects
mild diuretic helps use fat for
    energy
natural antidepressant
helps thyroid hormone action
normalizes blood clotting
helps normalize blood sugar
    levels
normalizes zinc and copper
    levels
maintains proper cell oxygen
    levels
protects against breast cysts
protects against breast cancer
protects against endometrial
    cancer
moisturizes skin when used
    topically,
counteracts estrogen side
    effects

Figure 20: The multiple roles of progesterone.

DHEA (Dehydroepiandrosterone)

DHEA is an adrenal-produced steroid hormone whose functions are not well known at this time despite the fact that it is produced in greater quantity than any other adrenal hormone. DHEA circulates in blood primarily as DHEA-S, a sulfated version which is not, in itself, biologically active. When blood tests for DHEA are done, the test results do not usually discriminate between the 95 percent which is DHEA-S and the 5 percent which is DHEA. Radioimmune assay of saliva, however, can be used to measure the concentration of the biologically active hormone, DHEA.

Plasma DHEA-S can be considered a circulating reservoir from which the active form can be derived. Conversely, DHEA can be converted back into DHEA-S. Regulators of this conversion process are not known. The enzymes that accomplish the conversions are known and are indicated in the diagram below.

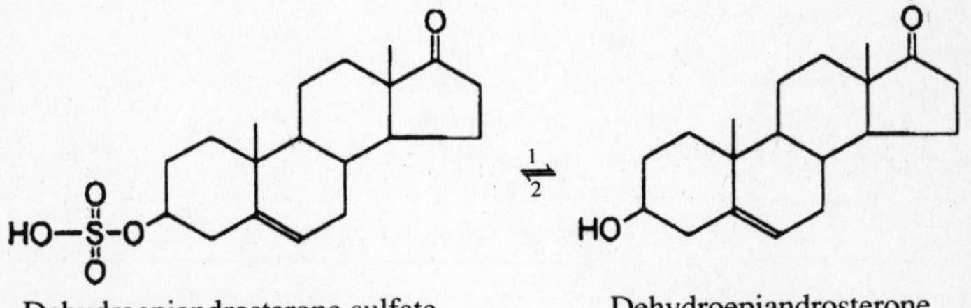

Dehydroepiandrosterone sulfate
DHEA-S

Dehydroepiandrosterone
DHEA

Figure 21: The enzymes that accomplish these transformations, labeled as 1 and 2 at the arrows, are the following:

1. *Sulfatases*
2. *Sulfokinases*

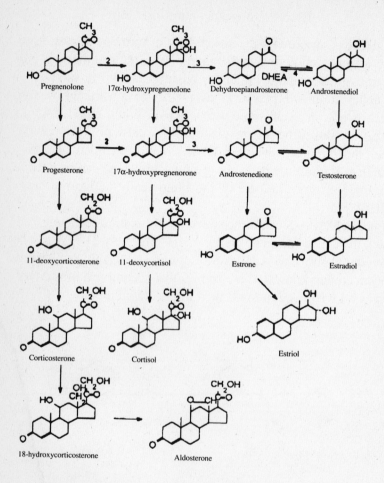

Figure 22: Steroidogenesis pathways.

INDEX

Crane's